Pathophysiology of the gut and airways

An introduction

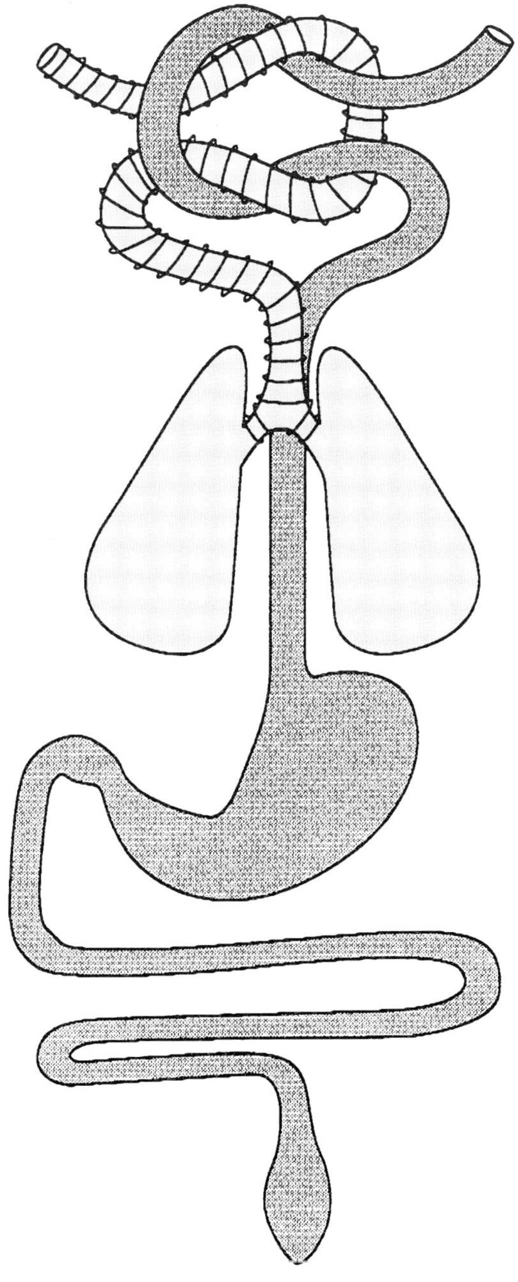

Pathophysiology of the gut and airways

An introduction

Editors
Paul Andrews
John Widdicombe

PORTLAND PRESS
London and
Chapel Hill

Published by Portland Press, 59 Portland Place,
London W1N 3AJ, U.K.
on behalf of the Physiological Society
In North America orders should be sent to Portland Press Inc.,
P.O. Box 2191, Chapel Hill, NC 27515-2191, U.S.A.

ISBN 1 85578 022 4 ISSN 0969-8116

British Library Cataloguing in Publication Data
A catalogue record for this book is available from
the British Library

Cover illustration by S. Bingham
Book design by A. Moyes

Typeset by Unicus Graphics Ltd, Horsham, Sussex
and Printed in Great Britain by Whitstable Litho Printers Ltd

Preface

The success of a Physiological Society symposium held at St George's Hospital Medical School, London, encouraged us to believe that there was a place for a short text introducing the growing subject of pathophysiology to a wide audience. The airways and gut were chosen as they are both interfaces with the outside environment and have a number of structural and functional similarities. In addition, both systems provide good examples of disorders where the underlying physiological defect is relatively well understood. By comparing aspects of normal and disordered physiology in the two systems we hope to encourage the reader to look for general principles as well as the detailed cellular mechanisms. To quote S. J. Gould from his book, *Wonderful Life*: "The beauty of nature lies in the detail; the message in generality".

Paul Andrews
John Widdicombe

Contents

1

Respiratory and gastro-intestinal parallels: real or contrived?

G. Burnstock
Department of Anatomy and Developmental Biology and Centre for Neuroscience, University College London, Gower Street, London WC1E 6BT, U.K.

Introduction

Since the lung is an embryological offshoot of the foregut, I would expect to see some basic similarities between these two organs. On the other hand, because the physiological roles of the gut and lung are diverse, I would also anticipate many differences. My task then is to make comparisons which highlight both the similarities and differences, and hopefully, through these comparisons, reveal some new avenues that will lead to a greater understanding of both systems.

Smooth muscle

Both the presence of smooth muscle bundles with gap-junctions providing low-resistance pathways between muscle cells, and the ultrastructural features of individual muscle cells, appear to be comparable in gut and airways [1, 2]. Muscle cells contain an abundance of contractile myofilaments and intermediate filaments that, together with dark bodies, form the structural framework. Smooth muscle cell membranes contain an abundance of caveolae alternating with dark areas forming attachment sites for myofilaments.

A striking feature of the muscle coats of the gut, however, is the presence of a complex network of cells, the interstitial cells of Cajal. These cells, which are innervated, form close contacts with each other and with smooth muscle cells and evidence is growing that they act as pacemakers for intestinal smooth muscle rhythmic activity [3, 4]. Some cells resembling interstitial cells have been described in the bronchial musculature (E. Daniel, personal communication) although these are considerably less numerous; their possible role as pacemakers has yet to be investigated.

Neuromuscular transmission

The relationship of autonomic nerves with smooth muscle is comparable in the two systems. The terminal regions of autonomic nerves consist of extensive branching varicose fibres. Transmitters are released from varicosities to reach receptors on smooth muscle membranes at distances varying from 20 nm to 1 or 2 μm [2, 5].

In the gastro-intestinal tract neuromuscular junctions are formed, not only by sympathetic and parasympathetic nerves, but also by projections from the enteric nervous system. Stimulation of the nerves to the non-sphincteric smooth muscle of the gut reveals the following:

— fast excitatory junction potentials in response to single stimuli which are due to acetylcholine (ACh);
— fast inhibitory junction potentials which are probably caused by ATP;
— slow hyperpolarizations in response to repetitive stimulation due to noradrenaline (NA);
— very slow non-adrenergic, non-cholinergic (NANC) relaxations and contractions caused by vasoactive intestinal polypeptide (VIP) and substance P (SP), respectively, in particular regions of the gastro-intestinal tract.

A variety of other substances, including neuropeptides, γ-amino butyric acid (GABA) and 5-hydroxytryptamine (5-HT) can modulate neuromuscular transmission in the gut [6, 7]. Recent studies [8, 9] suggest that nitric oxide (NO) might be a further NANC inhibitory transmitter, especially in sphincteric regions.

By comparison, in the smooth muscle of the airways, cholinergic excitatory innervation is present, NA-containing nerves seem to play a less prominent role in most species, and the nature of the NANC transmission is still unresolved. VIP is perhaps the strongest contender for slow NANC inhibitory responses [10, 11], but contributions from purines [12] and NO [13, 14] have also been claimed. A complication is that prostanoids, which are probably released as a consequence of transmitter action, also appear to contribute to the NANC responses [15, 16]. SP appears to be a potent NANC excitatory agent in the airways, and a role for calcitonin gene-related peptide (CGRP) released from sensory-motor nerves during axon-reflex activity must also be considered [17, 18].

The concept of co-transmission [19, 20] and of chemical coding [7], where the combinations of transmitters contained in neurons with projections to specific target sites and central connections have been identified, appears to apply equally to gastro-intestinal and airways systems. In particular, sympathetic nerves contain the combination of NA, ATP and neuropeptide Y (NPY), parasympathetic nerves contain ACh and VIP, and sensory-motor nerves contain SP and CGRP. Intrinsic NANC inhibitory neurons in gut and lung, containing variable proportions of VIP, ATP and NO, also appear to be present in both systems.

Intrinsic ganglia

Both gastro-intestinal and respiratory systems contain neurons located in intrinsic ganglia, although the intramural nervous system in the gut is clearly far larger and more complex than that found in the airways.

The enteric nervous system consists of two ganglionated plexuses, the myenteric (or Auerbach's) plexus lying between the longitudinal and circular muscle coats and the submucosal (or Meissner's) plexus. The neurons in these plexuses contain combinations of transmitters which project to different sites, including mucosal epithelial cells, smooth muscle cells and blood vessels, but many are interneurons involved in complex local reflect activities [7].

It is clear from recent studies that the intrinsic ganglia in the airways do not consist of simple parasympathetic nicotinic relay stations as was originally assumed, but rather involve an interneuronal and receptor complexity that is capable of sustaining integrative activity [21–23]. However, a key question remains: can the intrinsic neuronal circuitry within the airways sustain local reflex activity independent of the central nervous system as it clearly can in the gut?

- ► Smooth muscle cells are structurally similar in both gut and airways.
- ► Cells resembling the interstitial cells of Cajal in the gut have been described in the bronchial musculature; these are thought to act as 'pacemaker' cells.
- ► In both systems, transmitters are released from axon varicosities to the smooth muscle cells in an 'en passant' manner.
- ► The nature of the NANC transmission in particular regions of the gastro-intestinal tract has been established, whereas that in the smooth muscle of the airways is less well known.
- ► Co-transmission and the presence of neurons in intrinsic ganglia are features of the neurotransmission in both systems.

Blood vessels

The blood vessels in the gastro-intestinal tract and airways are controlled by a variety of co-transmitters released from sympathetic, parasympathetic, sensory-motor and intrinsic nerves [24]. However, the airway vasculature is unusual in that the majority of the bronchial blood drains into the pulmonary circulation and thence to the left side of the heart. The pulmonary and tracheobronchial circulations show a number of differences, in terms of both control and haemodynamic conditions. Whereas ischaemia and hypoxia cause vasodilation both in the gut and in the airways, they bring about vasoconstriction in the pulmonary bed. The vasculatures of both gut and airways have a neural control that is predominantly sympathetic inducing vasoconstriction mediated by NA and NPY; in addition there is a parasympathetic vasodilator modulation of vasomotor tone with ACh and VIP as the main neurotransmitters. Neurogenic inflammation, caused by axon reflexes in sensory nervous receptors releasing sensory neuropeptides, has been studied widely for the airways but less so for the gastro-intestinal tract. Neuropeptides such as SP, CGRP and neurokinin A (NKA) dilate both vascular beds [25]. Vasodilation of blood vessels in both gut and airways is mediated by endothelium-derived relaxing factors, probably consisting of both NO and prostanoids [26]. Vasoactive inflammatory agents including bradykinin, 5-HT, platelet-activating factor and ATP dilate both vascular beds [27]. The intrinsic neurons so well mapped out in the gut have not been clearly established for the airways but, if they exist there, their neurotransmitters might well have vascular actions.

► Epithelial secretion occurs in both systems and autonomic efferents and axon reflexes have been implicated in their control.
► The vasculature of both gut and airways is controlled predominantly by the sympathetic nervous system, but show a number of differences in terms of both control and haemodynamic conditions.
► A number of neuropeptides (e.g. SP, CGRP) and vasoactive inflammatory agents (e.g. bradykinin) dilate both vascular beds.
► Disorders of the autonomic control have been implicated in the pathophysiology of disease in both systems.

Epithelium

Mucosal epithelial cells in both the gastro-intestinal tract and lung show a plentiful supply of nerves at their bases, which arise from both intrinsic and extrinsic sensory and motor nerves [28, 29]. There is evidence for an epithelium-derived relaxing factor in the airways [30] but, as far as I am aware, this has not been revealed to date in the gut.

Other cells

A number of other cell types are involved in the physiology of gastro-intestinal and airways systems. Of particular importance in the lung are extra-adrenal medullary chromaffin [or SIF (small intensely fluorescent)] cells, neuro-epithelial bodies [31] and mast cells [32], which appear in large numbers in asthma patients.

Summary and conclusions

► Autonomic neural mechanisms that are common to the respiratory and gastro-intestinal systems are numerous.

► There are similarities in the nature of the autonomic neuroeffector junctions with the transmitters being released from varicosities to the smooth muscle cells, which are also structurally similar in the two systems.

► The multiplicity of neurotransmitters involved in the innervation of both the gut and the airways is notable, with peptides, purines, amino acids and, possibly, NO being implicated (see Chapters 2 and 3).

► In addition, co-transmission is a feature of the neurotransmission in both, as are pre- and post-junctional modulation of neuronal function.

► The airways and gut are both supplied with afferents projecting to the central nervous system and these have a multiplicity of functions including the activation of protective reflexes such as coughing (Chapter 10) and vomiting (Chapter 11), extrinsic reflects regulating motility and secretion, and 'axon reflexes' that may be involved in pathophysiological processes in both systems (Chapters 2 and 9).

► Although there are a number of similarities, each system also has many specialized features of structure and control.

► In the gut, the two most notable are the substantial network of interstitial cells (of Cajal) concerned with the pacemaker control of rhythmicity of the intestinal smooth muscle and the enteric nervous system located entirely within the walls of the gut that contains many millions of neurons (including sensory neurons); these provide the extensive and sophisticated circuitry needed to support the diverse range of complex local reflexes (Chapters 3 and 7).

► The specialized features of the respiratory system include the neural and/or endothelial mechanisms that facilitate hypoxic vasoconstriction, and the presence of an epithelium-derived relaxing factor.

References

1. Burnstock, G. (1970) Structure of smooth muscle and its innervation. In Smooth Muscle (Bülbring, E., Brading, A., Jones A and Tomita, T., eds.), pp. 1-69, Edward Arnold, London
2. Gabella, G. (1987) Innervation of airway smooth muscle: fine structure. Annu. Rev. Physiol. **49**, 583–594
3. Thuneberg, L. (1989) Interstitial cells of Cajal. In Handbook of Physiology: the Gastrointestinal System (Schultz, G. S., Wood, J. D. and Rauner, B. P., eds.), pp. 349–386, American Physiological Society, Bethesda
4. Barajas Lopez, C., Berezin, I., Daniel, E. E. and Huizinga, J. D. (1989) Pacemaker activity recorded in interstitial cells of Cajal of the gastrointestinal tract. Am. J. Physiol. **257**, C830–C835
5. Burnstock, G. (1986) Autonomic neuromuscular junctions: current developments and future directions. J. Anat. **146**, 1–30
6. Burnstock, G. (1986) The changing face of autonomic neurotransmission. (The First von Euler Lecture in Physiology). Acta Physiol. Scand. **126**, 67–91
7. Furness, J. B. and Costa, M. (1987) The Enteric Nervous System, Churchill Livingstone, Edinburgh
8. Bult, H., Boeckxstaens, G. E., Pelckmans, P. A., Jordaens, F. H., Van Maercke, Y. M. and Herman, A. G. (1990) Nitric oxide as an inhibitory non-adrenergic non-cholinergic neurotransmitter. Nature **345**, 346–347
9. Tottrup, A., Svane, D. and Forman, A. (1991) Nitric oxide mediating NANC inhibition in opussum lower esophageal sphincter. Am. J. Physiol. **260**, G385–G389
10. Venugopalan, C. S. (1989) Vasoactive intestinal peptide (VIP), a putative neurotransmitter of nonadrenergic, non-cholinergic (NANC) inhibitory innervation and its relevance to therapy. J. Vet. Pharmacol. Therapy **12**, 113–123
11. Ellis, J. L. and Farmer, S. G. (1989) The effects of vasoactive intestinal peptide (VIP) agonists, and VIP and peptide histidine isoleucine antisera on non-adrenergic, non-cholinergic relaxations of tracheal smooth muscle. Br. J. Pharmacol. **96**, 513–520
12. Satchell, D. (1982) Non-adrenergic, non-cholinergic nerves in mammalian airways: their function and the role of purines. Comp. Biochem. Physiol. **72C**, 189–196
13. Tucker, J. F., Brave, S. R., Charalambous, L., Hobbs, A. J. and Gibson, A. (1991) L-N^{G}-nitro arginine inhibits non-adrenergic, non-cholinergic relaxations of guinea-pig isolated tracheal smooth muscle. Br. J. Pharmacol. **100**, 663–664
14. Li, C. G., and Rand, M. J. (1991) Evidence that part of the NANC relaxant response of guinea-pig trachea to electrical field stimulation is mediated by nitric oxide. Br. J. Pharmacol. **102**, 91–94
15. De Jongste, J. C., Mons, H., Bonta, I. L. and Kerrebijn, K. F. (1987) Nonneuronal components in the response of fresh human airways to electric field stimulation. J. Appl. Physiol. **63**, 1558–1566
16. Regal, J. F. and Johnson, D. E. (1983) Indomethacin alters the effects of substance-P and VIP on isolated airway smooth muscle. Peptides **4**, 581–584
17. Maggi, C. A. and Meli, A. (1988) The sensory-efferent function of capsaicin-sensitive sensory nerves. Gen. Pharmacol. **19**, 1–43
18. Andersson, R. G. G. and Grundström, G. N. (1987) Innerviation of airway smooth muscle. Efferent mechanisms. Pharmacol. Therapeut. **32**, 107–130
19. Burnstock, G. (1976) Do some nerve cells release more than one transmitter? Neuroscience **1**, 239–248
20. Burnstock, G. (1990) Co-transmission. The Fifth Heymans Lecture — Ghent, February 17, 1990. Arch. Int. Pharmacodyn. Ther. **304**, 7–33
21. Coburn, R. F. (1987) Peripheral airway ganglia. Annu. Rev. Physiol. **49**, 573–582
22. Allen, T. G. J. and Burnstock, G. (1990) $GABA_A$ receptor-mediated increase in membrane chloride conductance in rat paratracheal neurones. Br. J. Pharmacol. **100**, 261–268
23. Allen, T. G. J. and Burnstock, G. (1990) A voltage-clamp study of the electrophysiological characteristics of the intramural neurones of the rat trachea. J. Physiol. (London) **423**, 593–614
24. Burnstock, G. (1990) Local mechanisms of blood flow control by perivascular nerves and endothelium. J. Hyperten. **8 (Suppl. 7)**, S95–S106
25. Salonen, R. O., Webber, S. E. and Widdicombe, J. G. (1990) Effects of neurotransmitters on tracheobronchial blood flow. Eur. Resp. J. **3 (Suppl. 12)**, 630S-637S
26. Rubanyi, G. M. (ed.) (1991) Cardiovascular Significance of Endothelium-Derived Vasoactive Factors, Futura, Mount Kisco, NY
27. Webber, S. E., Salonen, R. O., Corfield, D. R. and Widdicombe, J. G. (1990) Effects of non-neural mediators and allergen on tracheobronchial blood flow. Eur. Resp. J. **3 (Suppl. 12)**, 638S–644S
28. Laitinen, A. (1985) Ultrastructural organisation of intraepithelial nerves in the human airway tract. Thorax **40**, 488–492
29. Dey, R. D., Altemus, J. B., Zervos, I. and Hoffpauir, J. (1990) Origin and colocalization of CGRP- and SP-reactive nerves in cat airway epithelium. J. Appl. Physiol. **68**, 770–778
30. Flavahan, N. A., Aarhus, L. L., Rimele, T. J. and Vanhoutte, P. M. (1985) Respiratory epithelium inhibits bronchial smooth muscle tone. J. Appl. Physiol. **58**, 834–838
31. Lauweryns, J. M. and Van Lommel, A. (1987) Ultrastructure of nerve endings and synaptic junctions in rabbit intrapulmonary neuroepithelial bodies: a single and serial section analysis. J. Anat. **151**, 65–83
32. Guerzon, G. M., Paré, P. D., Michoud, M.-C. and Hogg, J. C. (1979) The number and distribution of mast cells in monkey lungs, Am. Rev. Respir. Dis. **119**, 59–66

2

Non-adrenergic non-cholinergic nerves in airways

Peter J. Barnes
Department of Thoracic Medicine, National Heart and Lung Institute, London SW3 6LY, U.K.

Introduction

Autonomic control of human airways is more complex than previously recognized, for, in addition to classic cholinergic and adrenergic pathways, neural mechanisms, which are neither cholinergic nor adrenergic, have been described [1, 2]. The existence of a non-adrenergic non-cholinergic (NANC) nervous system in the gastro-intestinal tract has long been established and, because the airways develop embryologically from the foregut, the presence of NANC nerves in airways is not surprising. Although NANC nerves in airways were originally conceived as a 'third' nervous system, it later became clear that NANC effects were mediated by several neurotransmitters. It now seems likely that there is no defined population of separate NANC nerves, but that NANC effects are mediated by the release of co-transmitters from 'classic' (i.e. adrenergic and cholinergic) autonomic nerves (Fig. 1). Some of these co-transmitters are neuropeptides and many different neuropeptides have now been localized to nerves in human and animal airways [3]. Neuropeptides may have potent effects on various aspects of airway function and there is increasing evidence that they may be involved in airway inflammatory diseases such as asthma.

For many centuries asthma has been viewed as an abnormality of the neural control of airways. There is a close interaction between the chronic inflammatory process in the airway wall and autonomic neural mechanisms. The recognition of NANC mechanisms, some of which are constrictor and proinflammatory and others of which are dilator and anti-inflammatory, has suggested that abnormal function of NANC nerves may be involved in asthma.

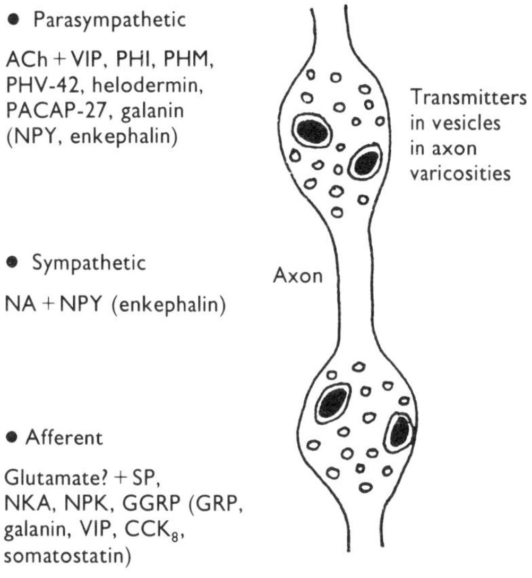

Fig. 1. Peptidergic co-transmission in airways
Numerous peptides are present in classic autonomic nerves of the airways which may function as co-transmitters and mediate NANC neuronal effects. Neuropeptides which are occasionally observed are shown in parentheses. Abbreviations used: ACh, acetylcholine; CCK_8, cholecystokinin octapeptide; CGRP, calcitonin gene-related peptide; GRP, gastrin-releasing peptide; NA, noradrenaline; NKA, neurokinin A; NPK, neuropeptide K; NPY, neuropeptide Y; PACAP-27, pituitary adenylate cyclase activating peptide; PHI, peptide histidine isoleucine; PHM, peptide histidine methionine; PHV-42, peptide histidine valine; SP, substance P; VIP, vasoactive intestinal polypeptide. Based on studies in a number of species.

Non-adrenergic inhibitory nerves

Inhibitory NANC (i-NANC) nerves, which relax airway smooth muscle, have been demonstrated *in vitro* in several species, including man [1, 2]. In human airway smooth muscle this i-NANC system is the only direct neural bronchodilator pathway, since there is no functional sympathetic innervation. Because NANC innervation appears to be the sole neural inhibitory pathway in human airway smooth muscle — from the trachea to the smallest bronchi — there has been particular interest in its physiological role and regulation, and speculation about whether its function might be impaired in asthma. NANC inhibitory nerves have also been demonstrated in animal airways *in vivo*, by electrical stimulation of the vagus nerve after cholinergic and adrenergic receptor blockade. Tantalum bronchography in cats shows that NANC bronchodilatation is predominantly seen in large airways. Stimulation of this pathway produces pronounced and long-lasting bronchodilatation and this response can be inhibited by ganglion blocking agents, suggesting that these NANC nerves are preganglionic (in addition to postganglionic nerves that can be demonstrated by field stimulation). It is not yet certain which physiological stimuli might activate this neural pathway, but mechanical stimulation of the larynx induces reflex NANC bronchodilatation in the cat. NANC nerves also mediate bronchodilatation in human airways *in vivo*, either stimulated by laryngeal irritation [4] or by inhalation of capsaicin [5]. In mild asthmatics there is no apparent defect in this i-NANC bronchodilator response [6].

NANC nerves also regulate secretion of airway mucus in animals [7]. Stimulation of the vagus nerves promotes mucus secretion in the cat trachea, which is reduced, but not abolished, by cholinergic and adrenergic blocking agents, and electrical field stimulation of ferret tracheal segments *in vitro* has shown NANC stimulation of mucus secretion.

The neurotransmitter of i-NANC nerves

Although it has been possible to demonstrate the existence of NANC nerves in the lung both *in vitro* and *in vivo*, it has proven difficult to investigate the physiological role of this component of the nervous system as the identity of the neurotransmitter(s) is still not certain and no specific antagonists are yet available. Purine receptors (e.g. ATP) have been implicated as neurotransmitters in the gastro-intestinal and genito-urinary tracts, and it has been suggested that non-adrenergic inhibitory nerves might therefore be purinergic. However, there is evidence which argues against a purine as the neurotransmitter of NANC nerves in the airways. Although exogenous ATP relaxes airway smooth muscle, an antagonist (quinidine) does not block NANC relaxation either *in vitro* or *in vivo*, nor does the purine uptake inhibitor dipyridamole enhance non-adrenergic bronchodilatation. Similarly, adenosine fails to mimic non-adrenergic relaxation and its antagonist theopylline does not block non-adrenergic relaxation.

Recent evidence suggests that nitric oxide (NO) may mediate NANC relaxation in several systems, such as bovine retractor penis, and preliminary evidence suggests that NO contributes to the i-NANC response in guinea-pig trachea, since nitroarginine, an inhibitor of NO synthesis, reduces the relaxation response induced by electrical field stimulation. In human airways, the NO synthesis inhibitor, N^{G}-monomethyl-L-arginine, similarly reduces the i-NANC response, particularly at low stimulus frequencies, and nitroarginine blocks most of the response, indicating that NO is a major transmitter.

Vasoactive intestinal polypeptide

Of the several peptides isolated from airways only vasoactive intestinal polypeptide (VIP) and a related peptide, peptide histidine isoleucine (PHI), relax airway smooth muscle [8]. VIP has been localized in both animal and human lungs to neurons and nerve terminals in airway smooth muscle (particularly in the upper airways), around submucosal glands, in the walls of bronchial and pulmonary vessels and in parasympathetic ganglia [3]. VIP produces prolonged relaxation of animal and human airway smooth muscle *in vitro*, which is unaffected by adrenergic or cholinergic blocking agents and mimics the electrophysiological changes in airway smooth muscle produced by NANC nerve stimulation. Inhaled VIP protects against histamine-induced bronchoconstriction *in vivo*, and reverses 5-hydroxytryptamine (5-HT)-induced bronchoconstriction in animals. In humans inhaled VIP has no bronchodilator effect in asthmatic patients who readily bronchodilate with an inhaled β-agonist, and it has only a weak protective effect against histamine-induced bronchoconstriction compared with a β-agonist. VIP has little or no bronchodilator effect when infused, despite profound cardiovascular effects. The relative lack of effect of VIP *in vivo* in humans may be explained by poor access of the relatively large peptide to its receptors in airway smooth muscle, by the fact that the cardiovascular effects limit the dose that can be infused, or by enzymic breakdown of the peptide by airway epithelium. The enzyme neutral endopeptidase (NEP) which is bound to airway epithelial cells appears to degrade VIP (see below).

VIP as i-NANC neurotransmitter

Electrical field stimulation of tracheal preparations releases VIP into the bathing medium and this is blocked by tetrodotoxin (a Na^+ channel blocker), indicating that VIP is derived from nerves. Furthermore, the amount of VIP released is related to the magnitude of the i-NANC response. Unfortunately, no specific blocker of VIP is yet available, but in cats prolonged incubation of airway smooth muscle with VIP reduces subsequent responses to VIP (tachyphylaxis or desensitization) and also reduces the magnitude of NANC nerve relaxation, while relaxation to sympathetic nerve stimulation and isoprenaline is unaffected. Preincubation of guinea-pig trachea with a specific antibody to VIP also reduces the i-NANC response. Incubation of guinea-pig trachea with the enzyme chymotrypsin, which degrades VIP, reduces but does not abolish the i-NANC response, although the enzyme may not reach sites of endogenous release of VIP. Selective phosphodiesterase inhibitors which potentiate the effect of VIP also enhance i-NANC relaxation in guinea-pig trachea. However, evidence against VIP is provided by the demonstration that incubation with maximally effective concentrations of VIP does not diminish i-NANC relaxation in guinea-pig trachea.

The distribution of VIP-ergic nerves in airways gives some clue to the role of VIP as a neutrotransmitter. Histochemical studies have demonstrated that the density of VIP-immunoreactive nerves diminishes in the small airways, and is virtually absent from bronchioles, and these small airways fail to relax in response to exogenous VIP, although they do relax with isoprenaline [9]. Taken together all this evidence points to VIP as a contributory neurotransmitter of i-NANC nerves, but conclusive proof, particularly in human airways, awaits the development of a potent and specific antagonist.

Other actions of VIP in airways

VIP-immunoreactive nerves are closely associated with airway submucosal glands and have complex effects on airway secretions [7]. VIP stimulates secretion of mucus from tracheal glands in the ferret *in vitro*, but this may depend on conditions of stimulation. VIP is therefore a plausible neurotransmitter for NANC secretion of mucus in this species. By contrast, VIP has an inhibitory effect on secretion of macromolecules from isolated human airways. VIP is also a potent stimulant of Cl^- transport and, therefore, water secretion across the epithelium in canine airways, although its effect on human airway epithelium is not known. Thus VIP-ergic nerves may regulate secretion of both mucus and water, and so influence mucociliary transport in the airways. VIP-ergic nerves may also modulate cholinergic neurotransmission in airways. VIP inhibits antigen-induced release of histamine from sensitized guinea-pig lung fragments *in vitro* and raises the possibility that VIP-ergic nerves may also regulate mast cell mediator secretion. Overall, VIP may be regarded as an anti-inflammatory peptide.

VIP receptors

VIP is released from nerve terminals and stimulates specific receptors, which have been demonstrated in lung membranes by radioligand-binding techniques with labelled VIP. Autoradiographic studies have shown that VIP receptors are widely distributed in human lung and are found in airway epithelium and submucosal glands, which suggests that VIP-ergic nerves may also regulate secretions in human airway [10]. Smooth muscle of large airways is also labelled, but that of peripheral airways is not, consistent with the finding that VIP relaxes bronchi, but not bronchioles.

VIP is a potent vasodilator and, in the tracheal circulation, may play an important role in the regulation of airway perfusion [11]. In the trachea, NANC vasodilator mechanisms of parasympathetic origin predominate, whereas neural control of the bronchial circulation seems to involve mainly afferent nerves [12]. VIP is more potent as a vasodilator in the tracheal than in the bronchial circulation, and may mediate vagally induced vasodilatation.

Co-transmission with acetylcholine

VIP-immunoreactive nerves are often distributed with cholinergic nerves. Ultrastructural studies suggest that VIP may exist in the same nerve terminals as acetylcholine and may, therefore, function as a co-transmitter [3]. It is possible that VIP, in addition to a direct effect on VIP receptors of target cells, may also have a prejunctional effect on acetylcholine release or an effect on postjunctional cholinergic receptors, as demonstrated in submaxillary glands. VIP reduces the contractile effect of exogenous acetylcholine on airway smooth muscle *in vitro*, but this does not appear to involve any change in muscarinic cholinergic receptor density or affinity, and may be due to a functional antagonism. Nevertheless, it is possible that physiologically VIP acts as a neuromodulator in airway smooth muscle, and it may be preferentially released under certain conditions. In the airways, VIP may be released only during intense vagal stimulation, acting as a braking mechanism. If this mechanism were deficient, it could result in exaggerated bronchoconstrictor responses, as seen in the bronchial hyper-responsiveness of asthma [13]. Another possible role for VIP could be as a regulator of bronchial blood flow, so that the blood supply to airway smooth muscle increases with cholinergic contraction.

Peptide histidine isoleucine

Peptide histidine isoleucine (PHI) has marked structural similarities to VIP and is coded by the same gene. PHI has an identical distribution in airways to that of VIP and also stimulates adenylate cyclase, probably via a specific receptor. PHI is a potent bronchodilator *in vitro*, being approximately equipotent to VIP, but is less potent as a vasodilator. It also stimulates airway mucus secretion. In humans, a related peptide, peptide histidine methionine (PHM) has been isolated and is as potent a relaxant of human bronchi *in vitro* as VIP. It is therefore probable that PHI/PHM is released with VIP and is also a neurotransmitter of non-adrenergic neural relaxation in the airways.

Abnormalities in asthma?

Whether dysfunction of i-NANC nerves may contribute to bronchial hyper-responsiveness in asthma is uncertain. *In vitro* there is no obvious relationship between the magnitude of NANC relaxation and the pre-operative responsiveness to inhaled histamine in patients with chronic obstructive pulmonary disease undergoing lobectomy, and no defect in NANC bronchodilator responses has been observed in mild asthmatic subjects [6]. It seems unlikely that there would be any primary defect in NANC innervation or in neuropeptide selective receptors, but it is possible that a functional defect in this system might develop as a result of the inflammatory process in the airway wall. Recently, an absence of VIP-immunoreactive nerves has been described in asthmatic lungs [14], although this might be due to post-mortem degradation of this peptide. Many enzymes may be released by the inflammatory cells which are involved in asthma (e.g. mast cells, neutrophils and eosinophils) which may break down VIP and PHI/PHM. This would be like inhibiting the braking mechanism due to VIP release from cholinergic nerves, and might result in exaggerated bronchoconstrictor responses [13] (Fig. 2). Mast cell tryptase is particularly effective in degrading VIP and high concentrations of tryptase have been demonstrated in bronchoalveolar lavage fluid in asthmatic patients.

- ► Inhibitory NANC nerves relax airway smooth muscle in several species; they also regulate secretion of airway mucus.
- ► NANC effects are mediated via a number of neurotransmitters, e.g. NO, VIP, PHI and PHM.
- ► The role of NANC effects in airway inflammatory disease, e.g. asthma, is uncertain, but abnormal function of i-NANC nerves may be a contributory factor.

Excitatory NANC nerves

Electrical stimulation of guinea-pig bronchi and trachea *in vitro* produces a component of bronchoconstriction which is not inhibited by atropine [15]. This excitatory NANC (e-NANC) response is mimicked by substance P (SP) and is inhibited by peptide analogues

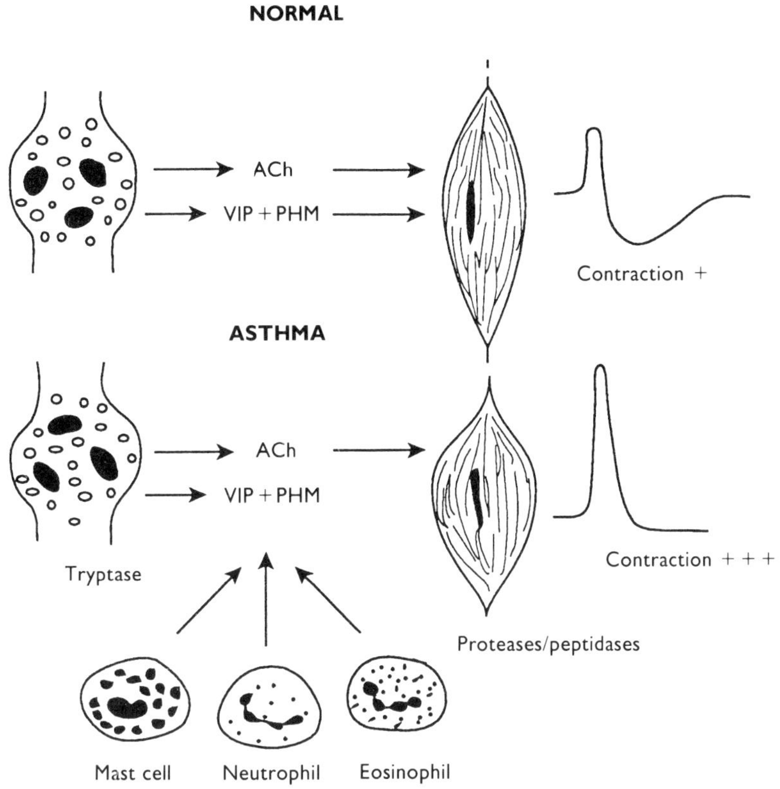

Fig. 2. VIP/PHM co-transmission in airway cholinergic nerves

VIP or PHM normally counteracts the constrictor effect of acetylcholine (ACh) on airway smooth muscle, but in asthma VIP and PHM are more rapidly degraded by enzymes such as tryptase released from mast cells, thus leading to enhanced cholinergic bronchoconstriction.

which are tachykinin antagonists, providing convincing evidence that SP and related tachykinins might be neurotransmitters of e-NANC nerves. Chronic capsaicin pretreatment, which destroys the sensory nerves which contain tachykinins and calcitonin gene-related peptide (CGRP), also blocks the e-NANC response. In human airways a non-cholinergic excitatory effect was found in only one out of eight airways tested, so that this neural mechanism may not be as easily demonstrable in normal human airways.

Substance P

SP is localized to non-myelinated sensory nerves (afferent C-fibres) in the airways of several species, including humans [16, 17]. There is evidence that SP-immunoreactive nerves may be increased in asthmatic airways [18]. SP-immunoreactive nerves in the airway are found beneath and within the airway epithelium, around blood vessels and, to a lesser extent, within airway smooth muscle. SP is synthesized in the nodose ganglion (the location of the cell bodies of the vagal afferents) of the vagus nerve and then transported down the vagus to peripheral branches in the lung. Treatment of animals with capsaicin releases SP from sensory nerves acutely, and chronic administration depletes the lung of SP. In man, inhalation of capsaicin induces cough and transient bronchoconstriction, which is seen in both normal and asthmatic subjects to an equal extent. SP infusion *in vivo* causes bronchoconstriction in animals; whereas in human subjects, while intravenous SP has profound cardiovascular effects, there is little effect on airway function; a small bronchoconstrictor response is followed by bronchodilatation at higher infusion doses. The cardiovascular actions may limit the dose that can be given and result in reflex bronchodilatation (by a reduction in vagal tone), which counteracts the bronchoconstriction. Even when given by inhalation SP has no significant effect on airway function in mild asthmatic subjects who are hyper-responsive to histamine given in the same way. This may be due to enzymic degradation of SP by the airway epithelium and its inability to cross the epithelium.

SP contracts airway smooth muscle of several species, including man *in vitro*. There is a high density of SP receptors on airway smooth muscle from trachea down to terminal bronchioles and this suggests that SP may be important in regulating the tone of peripheral airways. Moreover, capsaicin can induce a similar contraction, indicating release of SP from intrinsic nerves within airway smooth muscle. The contracile effect of SP on airway smooth muscle *in vitro* may be inhibited by SP receptor antagonists, suggesting a direct effect on smooth muscle cells, although the specificity of these antagonists has been questioned.

In rats and guinea-pigs, both SP and capsaicin induce oedema of the airway wall by increasing microvascular permeability. Depletion of SP nerves by neonatal capsaicin pretreatment prevents irritants, such as cigarette smoke and mechanical stimulation, from causing extravasation of plasma, suggesting that SP nerves mediate this effect. SP causes vasodilatation in the tracheobronchial circulation. SP is also a potent stimulant of airway mucus secretion in isolated canine airways and human airways [7, 19].

SP increases the release of mediators from rat peritoneal mast cells, and may be involved in the mediation of the wheal and flare response in the skin. SP injected intradermally in man produces a wheal which is blocked by antihistamines and increases the release of histamine into draining veins. SP does not appear to cause direct degranulation of airway mast cells, however. Thus, SP could account for many of the pathological changes seen in asthma, including:

— contraction of airway smooth muscle
— bronchial wall oedema
— extravasation of plasma
— mucus hypersecretion
— increased release of mediators from inflammatory cells.

In addition, it has been postulated that SP might amplify neutrophil and eosinophil responses to chemotactic agents, and therefore magnify the inflammatory response in the airways.

Other tachykinins

In some tissues SP is more potent (NK-1 receptor), whereas in others the related tachykinin which may be coded by the same gene, neurokinin A (NKA), is more potent (NK-2 receptor). NKA is more potent than SP in contracting airway smooth muscle *in vitro* and *in vivo*, suggesting that receptors on airway smooth muscle are of the NK-2 subtype. By contrast, SP is more potent than NKA in causing airway microvascular leak, vasodilatation and mucus secretion, indicating that NK-1 receptors are involved in these responses.

Enzymic degradation

Removal of the epithelium potentiates the bronchoconstrictor effects of several spasmogens, but this is particularly marked for tachykinins. For NKA this can be explained by the fact that neural endopeptidase (NEP) is localized in airway epithelium and, in the presence of an NEP inhibitor, no effect of epithelial removal is seen [20]. For SP it is more complex, since SP also appears to release relaxant factors, including prostaglandins, from airway epithelium via NK-1 receptors. Epithelium shedding occurs in asthma and this means that tachykinins released from sensory nerves will not be rapidly degraded in the absence of epithelial NEP. This may result in increased tachykinin effects, not only on airway smooth muscle but also (and perhaps more importantly) on microvascular leakage, airway blood flow and mucus secretion (Fig. 3). Inhibition of NEP by drugs such as phosphoramidon and thiorphan greatly potentiates the effects of SP and NKA and of e-NANC nerve stimulation.

Calcitonin gene-related peptide

Another peptide which is localized to sensory nerves is CGRP, a 37-amino-acid peptide which may be co-stored and co-released with SP [16]. CGRP has no consistent effects on guinea-pig

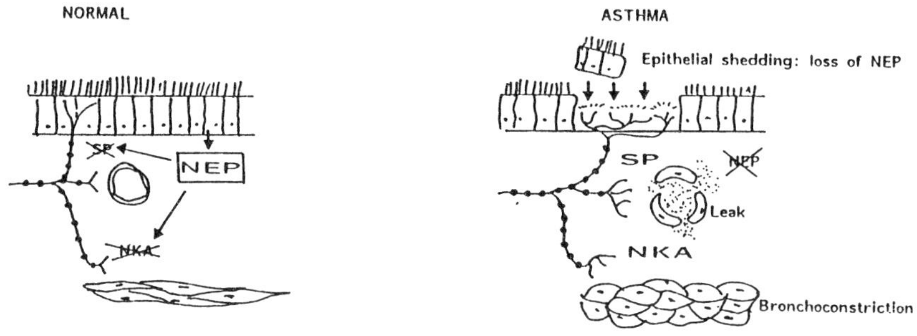

Fig. 3. Effect of tachykinins in asthma
NEP expressed on airway epithelium normally degrades any NKA released from sensory nerves. If epithelium is shed or NEP is down-regulated (as may occur in asthma) any tachykinins released from sensory nerves may have an exaggerated effect.

airways, but contracts human airways *in vitro*. It has potent effects on vascular smooth muscle, and also produces a long-lasting flare in human skin when injected locally [21].

CGRP is a very potent dilator of bronchial vessels, both *in vivo* and *in vitro* [11]. Autoradiographic mapping studies have shown that CGRP-receptors are localized predominantly on bronchial vessels in animal and human airways [22]. This suggests that CGRP may be an important regulator of bronchial blood flow and may be responsible for the hyperaemia of inflamed airways in asthma. CGRP does not cause microvascular leakage in airways, but could theoretically enhance SP-induced leakage by increasing the blood flow to leaky vessels. Ekström et al. [23] observed a similar modulation with SP-induced salivary secretion, although CGRP had no effect on resting output.

Axon reflexes

Antidromic release of neuropeptides from sensory nerves may lead to local inflammation. Because sensory neuropeptides SP, NKA and CGRP produce many of the pathological features of asthma, it is possible that they may be involved in the pathology of asthma. Damage to airway epithelium may occur even in relatively well-controlled asthmatics, exposing afferent nerve endings which are stimulated by inflammatory mediators. C-fibre endings may be selectively stimulated by bradykinin and prostaglandins produced in the inflammatory reaction, which could result in a reflex cholinergic bronchoconstriction. However, anticholinergic drugs are not very effective in clinical asthma and it is possible that stimulation of C-fibre endings may also result in an axon reflex, with release of sensory neuropeptides from sensory collaterals in the airway [24]. In addition, local ganglion reflexes may be activated, and SP-immunoreactive nerve terminals may be seen around human airway ganglia. The release of SP, neurokinins and CGRP may then result in bronchoconstriction, mucus hypersecretion and microvascular leakage of plasma to produce oedema of the airway wall and extravasation of plasma into the airway lumen (Fig. 4). The axon reflex may, therefore, amplify and spread the inflammation in asthmatic airways. It may be enhanced in asthma by a loss of NEP from shed epithelial cells or by down-regulation of NEP, and by a proliferation of SP-immunoreactive nerves.

There is still little direct evidence for the involvement of axon reflex mechanisms in human asthma, although direct evidence would be difficult to obtain. In experimental animals evidence suggests that capsaicin-sensitive nerves participate in some allergic responses. Thus, depletion of these nerves by pretreatment with capsaicin reduces the vasodilator response to allergen in pig airways. Both sensory denervation and a tachykinin antagonist appear to inhibit the increased airway responsiveness which follows exposure of guinea-pigs to toluene di-isocyanate.

Modulation of e-NANC nerve activity

e-NANC nerve activity may be modulated by a number of pharmacological agents which

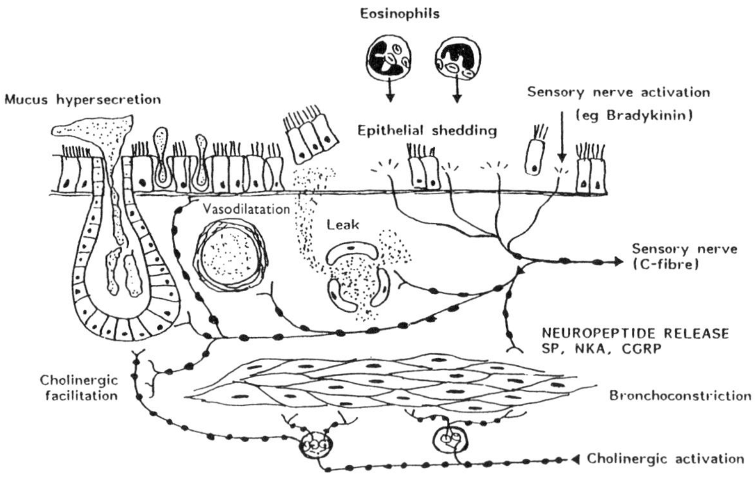

Fig. 4. Neurogenic inflammation in asthma
Activation of exposed and sensitized sensory nerve endings may lead to release of neuropeptides from collateral branches, which will amplify the ongoing inflammatory response. Thus, SP will cause microvascular leak, vasodilatation and mucus secretion, whereas NKA will cause bronchoconstriction and enhanced cholinergic neurotransmission, and CGRP will cause prolonged vasodilatation.

include opioids (via μ-opioid receptors), γ-aminobutyric acid (GABA) (via $GABA_B$ receptors), neuropeptide Y, α_2 receptor agonists and histamine H_3-receptor agonists [25]. These prejunctional inhibitory receptors could work through a similar mechanism, such as the opening of a common potassium channel.

Other drugs may prevent the activation of airway sensory nerves. The anti-asthma drugs, sodium cromoglycate and nedocromil sodium, appear to have inhibitory effects on neurogenic responses, perhaps by preventing neural activation.

► The eNANC response (atropine-resistant bronchoconstriction) is mimicked by SP and inhibited by tachykinin antagonists, suggesting a role for SP and sensory neuropeptides (NKA; CGRP) as neurotransmitters of eNANC nerves.
► Release of sensory neuropeptides (e.g. via the axon reflex) may lead to local inflammation which is amplified and spread in asthmatic airways.
► Sensory neuropeptides may account for some of the pathological features seen in asthma.

Conclusions

► NANC mechanisms in airways regulate airway tone, secretions and blood flow, and may modulate the inflammatory response.

► It has proven difficult to study NANC mechanisms in normal and asthmatic humans *in vivo*, however, in the absence of specific antagonists.

► Development of potent and specific antagonists of neuropeptide receptors has proven to be extraordinarily difficult, although recently more useful compounds have been emerging.

► It seems likely that NANC mechanisms may normally be involved in 'fine tuning' of the classical autonomic control, and may play an important role in airway diseases such as asthma [26].

► In the future the application of molecular biological probes to investigate factors regulating synthesis of neuropeptides may shed new light on their role in disease.

I thank Madeleine Wray for her careful preparation of the manuscript.

References

1. Richardson, J. B. (1981) Nonadrenergic inhibitory innervation of the lung. Lung **159**, 315–322
2. Barnes, P. J. (1986) State of art. Neural control of human airways in health and disease. Am. Rev. Resp. Dis. **134**, 1289–1314
3. Uddman, R. and Sundler, F. (1987) Neuropeptides in the airways: a review. Am. Rev. Resp. Dis. **136**, S3–8
4. Michoud, M.-C., Amyot, R., Jeanneret-Grosjean, A. and Couture, J. (1987) Reflex decrease of histamine-induced bronchoconstriction after laryngeal stimulation in humans. Am. Rev. Resp. Dis. **136**, 618–622
5. Lammers, J.-W., Minette, P., McCusker, M. T., Chung, K. F. and Barnes, P. J. (1988) Nonadrenergic bronchodilator mechanisms in normal human subjects *in vivo*. J. Appl. Physiol. **64**, 1817–1822
6. Lammers, J.-W., Minette, P., McCusker, M. T., Chung, K. F. and Barnes, P. J. (1989) Capsaicin-induced bronchodilation in asthmatic patients: role of the nonadrenergic inhibitory system. J. Appl. Physiol. **67**, 856–861
7. Webber, S. E. (1990) Nonadrenergic noncholinergic control of mucus secretion in airways. Arch. Int. Pharmacodyn. **303**, 100–112
8. Barnes, P. J., Baronivk, J. and Belvisi, M. G. (1991) State of the art. Neuropeptides in the respiratory tract. Am. Rev. Resp. Dis. **144**, 1187–1198; 1391–1399
9. Palmer, J. B., Cuss, F. M. C. and Barnes, P. J. (1986) VIP and PHM and their role in non-adrenergic inhibitory responses in isolated human airways. J. Appl. Physiol. **61**, 1322–1328
10. Carstairs, J. R. and Barnes, P. J. (1986) Visualization of vasoactive intestinal peptide receptors in human and guinea pig lung. Pharmacol. Exp. Therapeut. **248**, 292–299
11. Widdicombe, J. G. (1990) The NANC system and airway vasculature. Arch. Int. Pharmacodyn. **303**, 83–90
12. Matran, R., Alving, K., Martling, C.-R., Lacroix, J. S. and Lundberg, J. M. (1989) Vagally mediated vasodilation by motor and sensory nerves in the tracheal and bronchial circulation of the pig. Acta Physiol. Scand. **135**, 29–37
13. Barnes, P. J. (1991) Neuropeptides and asthma. Am. Rev. Resp. Dis. **143**, S28–S32
14. Ollerenshaw, S., Jarvis, D., Woolcock, A., Sullivan, C. and Scheibner, T. (1989) Absence of immunoreactive vasoactive intestinal polypeptide in tissue from the lungs of patients with asthma. N. Engl. J. Med. **320**, 1244–1248
15. Andersson, R. G. G. and Grundstrom, N. (1983) The excitatory non-cholinergic, non-adrenergic nervous system of the guinea-pig airways. Eur. J. Resp. Dis. **64**, 141–157
16. Lundberg, J. M., Saria, A., Lundblad, L., Angaard, A., Martling, C.-R., Theodorsson-Norheim, E., Stjarne, P. and Hokfelt, T. (1987) Bioactive peptides in capsaicin-sensitive C-fiber afferents of the airways: functional and pathophysiological implications. In The Airways: Neural Control in Health and Disease (Kaliner, M. A. and Barnes, P. J., eds), pp. 417–445, Marcel Dekker, New York
17. Barnes, P. J. (1990) Neurogenic inflammation in airways and its modulation. Arch. Int. Pharmacodyn. **303**, 67–82
18. Ollerenshaw, S. L., Jarvis, D. L., Woolcock, A. J., Scheibner, T. and Sullivan, C. E. (1991) Substance P immunoreactive nerve fibres in airways from patients with and without asthma. Eur. Resp. J. **4**, 673–682
19. Rogers, D. F., Aursudkij, B. and Barnes, P. J. (1989) Effects of tachykinins on mucus secretion in human bronchi *in vitro*. Eur. J. Pharmacol. **174**, 283–286
20. Frossard, N., Rhoden, K. J. and Barnes, P. J. (1989) Influence of epithelium on guinea pig airway responses to tachykinins: role of endopeptidase and cyclooxygenase. J. Pharmacol. Exp. Therapeut. **248**, 292–299
21. Brain, S. D., Williams, T. J., Tippins, J. R., Morris, H. R. and MacIntyre, I. (1985) Calcitonin gene-related peptide is a potent vasodilator. Nature (London) **313**, 54–56
22. Mak, J. C. M. and Barnes, P. J. (1988) Autoradiographic localization of calcitonin gene-related peptide binding sites in human and guinea pig lung. Peptides **9**, 957–964
23. Ekstrom, J., Ekman, R., Hakanson, R., Sjogren, S. and Sundlor, F. (1988). Calcitonin gene-related peptide in cat salivary glands: neuronal localization, depletion upon nerve stimulation, and effects of salivation in relation to substances. Neuroscience **26**, 933–949
24. Barnes, P. J. (1986) Asthma as an axon reflex. Lancet i, 242–245
25. Barnes, P. J., Belvisi, M. G. and Rogers, D. F. (1990) Modulation of neurogenic inflammation: novel approaches to inflammatory diseases. Trends Pharmacol. Sci. **11**, 185–189
26. Barnes, P. J. (1989) Airway neuropeptides: roles in fine tuning and in disease. News Physiol. Sci. **4**, 116–120

3

Non-adrenergic non-cholinergic motor systems in the gastro-intestinal tract

G. J. Sanger
SmithKline Beecham Pharmaceuticals, Coldharbour Road, The Pinnacles, Harlow, Essex CM19 5AD, U.K.

Introduction

Until recent years, research within the enteric nervous system focused almost entirely on those systems which used acetylcholine (ACh) and noradrenaline (NA) as neurotransmitters. However, after an initial period of controversy, it is now accepted that other substances can also act as neurotransmitters. These have important roles within gastro-intestinal motility and secretion mechanisms (see Chapter 7) in both health and disease; they act as neuromodulators and, in some circumstances, as the final mediator of neuronal control. The growing recognition of the importance of the different neurotransmitters within the enteric nervous system has already led to the identification of novel targets for new drug development. Such a trend is likely to continue. This chapter is therefore intended to provide a brief overview of some of the major physiological and pathophysiological functions of neurotransmitters other than ACh and NA within the enteric nervous system.

The enteric nervous system

Between the different layers of tissue comprising the gut wall are eight different nerve plexuses [1]. There are also nerves associated with the vasculature. Of the nerve plexuses, the myenteric (Auerbach's) and submucosal (Meissner's) are the most prominent and have been most often studied and linked to gut functions. The myenteric plexus lies between the outer longitudinal and inner circular muscle. It is associated with the overall control of gut motility. The submucosal plexus lies below the circular muscle and within the submucosa. Its function is associated with the modulation of gastric and intestinal secretions and with fluid and ion absorption from the lumen of the gut (see Chapter 7). However, it is important to appreciate that each of the nerve plexuses are interconnected, so that stimuli which affect fluid secretion and absorption can also evoke a corresponding change in gut motility, and *vice versa.*

Gut nerves may contain and, when activated, release one or more substances. Depending on their action, these have been variously described as neurotransmitters, neuromodulators (affecting the action of a neurotransmitter) or as trophic factors (affecting the growth or metabolism of cells). However, a simpler approach is to describe as neurotransmitters all substances that are released from nerve endings under physiological conditions, to affect a direct or indirect action on the target cell [2].

The most important criteria for identification of a substance as a neurotransmitter are that its release from a nerve must be detected and that the action of the substance released by nerve stimulation can be mimicked by its exogenous application.

These criteria are greatly strengthened if an antagonist can be used to selectively block the activity of both the exogenously applied and endogenously released substance [1]. Table 1 lists the substances proposed as neurotransmitters in the gut, many of which are peptides [3]. A critical assessment of the merits of these proposals can be found in [1]. Some of these substances are co-localized within the same nerve terminal, or even within the same vesicles [4]. For example, Bornstein and Furness [5] identified four types of submucous neurons in guinea-pig ileum:

— 'cholinergic secretomotor neurons' (as described using functional assays), when

Table 1 **Proposed enteric neurotransmitters**

Peptides	Non-peptides
Angiotensin II	Acetylcholine (ACh)
Angiotensin I	Noradrenaline (NA)
Calcitonin gene-related peptide (CGRP)	5-hydroxytryptamine (5-HT)
Cholecystokinin 8	γ-aminobutyric acid (GABA)
Dynorphin A	Adenosine triphosphate (ATP)
Leu-enkephalin	
Met-enkephalin	
Galanin	
Gastrin-releasing peptide	
Neuropeptide Y	
Neurotensin	
Peptide HI	
Somatostatin	
Substance K (neurokinin A)	
Substance P	
Thyrotropin-releasing hormone	
Vasoactive intestinal peptide (VIP)	

examined by histochemistry were found to contain choline-acetyltransferase (ChAT), calcitonin gene-related peptide (CGRP), cholecystokinin, neuropeptide Y, somatostatin and, usually, galanin

— 'non-cholinergic secretomotor neurons' contained dynorphin, galanin and vasoactive intestinal peptide (VIP)

— 'cholinergic interneurons' contained ChAT alone

— nerves thought to be sensory contained ChAT and substance P (SP).

The same neurotransmitter may, therefore, be present within two groups of functionally different neurons, which may even interconnect (intrinsic interneurons and afferent or efferent neurons). Although these combinations of neuropeptides and 'classical' neurotransmitters are found in the submucous plexus of the guinea-pig, it is important to realize that they may be present in other combinations in different locations or even the same location in other species. Studies of the 'rules' governing the various combinations and the functional implications of such combinations are in their infancy.

The release of each individual co-localized neurotransmitter cannot be differentially regulated by individual autoreceptors. However, the type of neurotransmitter released might be regulated by the intensity and frequency of stimulation, or by chronic drug treatment. Furthermore, stores of some neurotransmitters are easily replenished during repetitive stimulation, whereas for others (e.g. peptides) the rate of re-synthesis is slow. Since the action of one neurotransmitter can be modulated by another, the consequences of a small variation in the release of a modulating neurotransmitter can be greatly amplified. The system is therefore geared for maximum sensitivity to change.

Non-adrenergic, non-cholinergic-mediated responses

Within the gastro-intestinal tract, many different neuronally mediated responses have been described, which are not blocked by drugs that prevent cholinergic and noradrenergic function. Such responses have been ascribed to activation of non-adrenergic, non-cholinergic (NANC) enteric excitatory or inhibitory neurons. However, because neurotransmitters are usually co-localized, this definition must be treated with caution. For example, in the presence of the muscarinic receptor antagonist atropine, a neuronally mediated response may be due to the release of a substance from a nerve which also contains acetylcholine (ACh).

The nerve could, therefore, be described as both 'cholinergic' and 'non-cholinergic'. For this reason, although we will use the conventional abbreviation of 'NANC', only non-ACh or non-noradrenaline (NA)-mediated responses will be discussed, as this does not make an unwarranted assumption about the neurochemical nature of the neuron involved.

Most early descriptions of NANC-mediated responses do not attribute physiological function to the responses measured [1]. A typical example is shown in Fig. 1. In this experiment, electrical field stimulation of human isolated stomach evokes a longitudinal muscle contraction. This occurs because the electrical current simultaneously activates all of the intrinsic neurons but, because the cholinergic fibres dominate, a contraction is evoked. However, by preventing the action of ACh with atropine, the same electrical stimulation now evokes a muscle relaxation which cannot be antagonized by a mixture of adrenoceptor antagonists. The relaxation is therefore said to be caused by the activation of NANC inhibitory neurons.

In this chapter, discussion of NANC-mediated responses is limited to those areas in which a function can be ascribed. Particular emphasis is placed on the ability of the intrinsic nerves of the gut to control their own environment in response to food or to noxious events. Limited discussion is given to the large part also played by neurotransmitters other than ACh and NA in the signalling of information to the spinal cord, spinal ganglia and brain. By such pathways, one region of the gut can also signal to another, modulate gut motility and co-ordinate intestinal function with extra-intestinal functions, such as pancreatic and biliary secretion [6].

- ► Substances other than ACh and NA can act as neurotransmitters, particularly within the enteric nervous system.
- ► The same neurotransmitter may be present within two groups of functionally different neurons
- ► Because neurotransmitters are usually co-localized, the definition of 'NANC' should be used with caution; e.g. a NANC

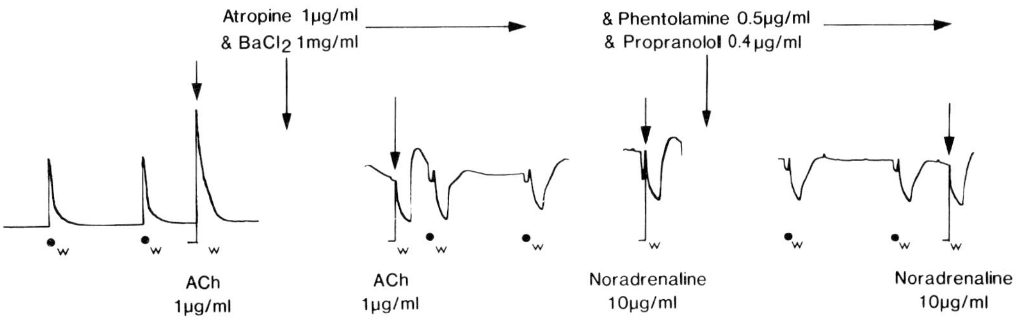

Fig. 1. Cholinergic and NANC inhibitory responses in human isolated stomach

In this experiment, a section of stomach wall (with mucosa and submucosa removed) was cut parallel to the outer longitudinal uscle layers. When suspended in a tissue bath, electrical field stimulation (●; 5 Hz frequency, bipolar rectangular pulses of 1 ms width, 160 V/cm, 30 s duration) evoked a contraction which was subsequently prevented by the addition of atropine (1 µg/ml) to the bathing solution. When the tone of the muscle was raised by the addition of BaCl (100 µg/ml) to the bath, the same electrical stimulation could now be seen to evoke a muscle relaxation, resistant to adrenoceptor blockade by phentolamine (0.5 µg/ml) plus propranolol (0.4 µg/ml). Responses to drugs are highlighted by vertical bars. In additional experiments (not shown here), both the excitatory and inhibitory responses to these parameters of electrical stimulation can be prevented by tetrodotoxin (1 µg/ml). The responses illustrated by this experiment are, therefore, due to activation of cholinergic excitatory neurons and NANC inhibitory neurons. While this type of experiment played an important role in first identifying and then characterizing NANC neurons, it does not provide any information on their function. Abbreviation used: W, wash.

response may be due to the release of a substance from a nerve which also contains ACh (e.g. VIP and ACh are often co-localized in neurons).

Physiological significance of non-adrenergic, non-cholinergic neuronal activity

The gut must detect and respond to events which occur within its own lumen. A bolus of food will therefore activate several different mechanoreceptors (rapidly adapting, slowly adapting, etc.) contained within different layers of the gut wall and, depending on its composition, chemoreceptors. As a result, the following events may be initiated to accommodate, move and, where appropriate, absorb the food.

1. Accommodation

During the continued presence of constant stretch the circular muscle of guinea-pig or human isolated colon slowly increases in length, overcoming the normal property of stretched smooth muscle to depolarize. This reflex, known as 'accommodation', has particular relevance to the storage function of the colon, and does not occur in the ileum [1].

In the stomach, accommodation of the fundus is also an important mechanism by which food is stored, before entering the pylorus for mixing and propulsion into the duodenum. However, unlike the colon, intrinsic nerves may play little or no role in initiating the reflex. Instead muscle relaxation is achieved by a vago-vagal reflex activating an inhibitory nerve which utilizes a transmitter other than ACh or NA (see [1] for references). Such pathways also modulate antral motility and indirectly control gastric tone as a result of oesophageal or duodenal distension.

Where studied, the final intrinsic neurotransmitter involved in accommodation may be VIP, although it should be stressed that this may not be true of all species or gut regions [1, 7].

2. Ascending excitation and descending inhibition

In the circular muscle of the small intestine, bolus distension, radial stretching or chemical stimuli applied to the mucosa activate mechano- and/or chemoreceptors to cause a contraction above (orally) the point of stimulus (enteric ascending excitatory reflex) and a relaxation below (anally) the stimulus (enteric descending inhibitory reflex). The pathways of these reflexes are illustrated in Fig. 2. They influence the entire circumference of the gut and transmit information to the longitudinal muscle for appropriate co-ordination. The length of the ascending excitatory response may vary from 4 to 10 cm, depending on the species. This is achieved by short (1 mm) axons projecting to additional excitatory neurons both in an oral direction and circumferentially. The descending inhibitory response may vary from 1 to 2 cm up to 14 cm, involving an unknown number of interneurons and a final neuron that evokes an inhibitory response mediated by a transmitter other than ACh or NA (see [1, 7]).

The above ascending and descending enteric reflexes are essential, individual components of the peristaltic reflex. By this mechanism a bolus is 'pushed' down the intestine by the excitatory response, being received by a relaxed segment of intestine with a correspondingly reduced resistance to flow. However, by electrically stimulating the myenteric plexus, an additional excitatory nerve pathway, projecting anally, has been described. The function of this pathway is not clear, but it could be involved in limiting the duration of the descending inhibitory pathway, or in the mechanisms of retropulsion. Propagation of an intraluminal bolus is, therefore, dependent on the continued activation of the peristaltic reflex as it passes down the gut. If the bolus is allowed to exit through an opening, the peristaltic wave stops.

The final excitatory and inhibitory neurons involved in the peristaltic reflex originate within the myenteric plexus and supply the circular muscle. This is demonstrated simply by experiments with isolated gut tissue, in which NANC-mediated inhibitory and excitatory responses are more readily demonstrated in circular, rather than in the longitudinal muscle preparations used to illustrate Fig. 1.

Excitatory neurotransmitters

In general, ACh is the predominant neurotransmitter involved in the ascending excitatory reflex. In some tissues, SP or a related tachykinin (substance K) may also be involved. For these tissues, the cholinergic neurons are

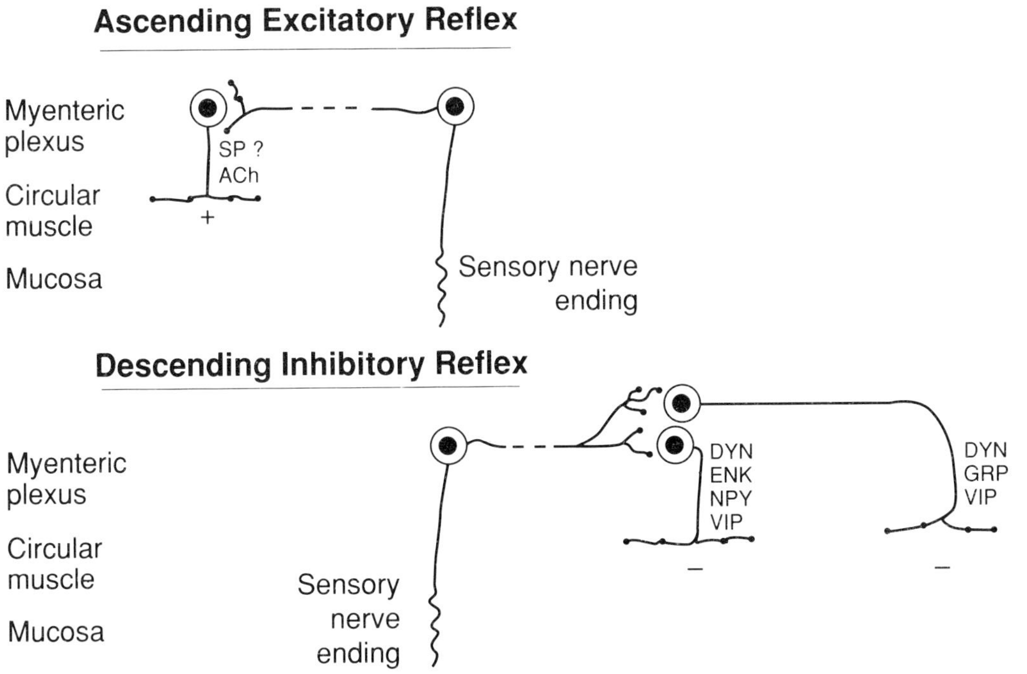

Fig. 2. Simplified diagram to show the major neuronal pathways involved in the ascending excitatory and descending inhibitory reflexes within the guinea-pig ileum, both of which are major components of the peristaltic reflex

In each case, the sensory nerve ending is shown as originating from within the mucosa, although it should be appreciated that these pathways can also be activated via activation of nerve terminals deeper within the gut wall. The connections between the sensory fibres and the motor neurons are depicted as broken lines, since it is not yet known whether the connection is made directly or via an interneuron. In each case, the motor neurons contain a number of different neurotransmitters. Abbreviations used: ACh, acetylcholine; DYN, dynorphin; ENK, enkephalin; GRP, gastrin-releasing peptide; NPY, neuropeptide Y; SP, substance P; VIP, vasoactive intestinal polypeptide.

activated by low threshold stimuli, whereas the SP-containing neurons require higher grades of stretch before they are activated. Alternatively, ACh and SP may co-exist in the same neuron with the release of each substance being controlled by the 'intensity' or frequency of nerve firing [8]. ACh may, therefore, be involved primarily in the initial ascending excitatory reflex, whereas SP may play a role in maintaining the reflex (where necessary) and/or in defence mechanisms which protect the gut from painful noxious events (e.g. the retrograde peristalsis of vomiting; see Chapter 11). It has been speculated that these roles might even be interchangeable, providing considerable scope for protecting the function of peristalsis. Whether this proposed role for SP is also applicable in tissues where an alternative peptide (e.g. enkephalins) may serve as the neurotransmitter is not known.

The neurotransmitters mediating the descending excitatory pathway (evoked by electrical nerve stimulation) may be 5-hydroxytryptamine (5-HT) [acting on 5-HT sub-type 3 (5-HT_3) receptors] and ACh in guinea-pig ileum [9] or an opiate and ACh in dog intestine [10].

Inhibitory neurotransmitters

The neurotransmitter involved in the descending inhibitory reflex may, in some species and gut regions, be VIP and/or the related substances peptide histidine isoleucine (PHI) or peptide histidine methionine (PHM) [11]. Of these peptides VIP is likely to dominate, since the related peptides are less potent and less stable [8].

The involvement of VIP has been demonstrated using circular muscle preparations of rat and guinea-pig colon, human jejunum and guinea-pig ileum. Responses were evoked by graded radial stretch of whole intestine or by electrical field stimulation of the myenteric plexus, and were blocked by receptor desensitization, VIP receptor antagonists or antiserum. In addition, the ascending excitatory response is increased by VIP antiserum, implying that a background release of VIP exerts a tonic influence on the entire peristaltic reflex [8]. However, it is important to appreciate that neurotransmitters other than VIP may mediate the NANC-mediated inhibitory responses in at least some species and/or gut regions. Examples of alternative candidates include the adenosine compounds (e.g. ATP) and CGRP.

Modulation of ascending and descending reflexes

The ascending and/or inhibitory reflex may be modulated by both sympathetic neurons and NANC-mediated nerve activity. For example, opioid peptides inhibit VIP release in rat colon. Opioid release is decreased during peristalsis, thereby reducing a constraining influence on the descending inhibitory reflex in the circular muscle and on cholinergic excitatory fibres in the longitudinal muscle [8]. Furthermore, VIP release may be increased by somatostatin and decreased by somatostatin antiserum, implying that in this tissue, somatostatin-containing myenteric neurons act as facilitatory interneurons in descending pathways, perhaps by suppressing opiate-containing nerve activity. On this basis it has been suggested that a peristaltic stimulus activates somatostatin-containing neurons reducing opiate release and increasing VIP release [8].

With regards to the ascending excitatory reflex, the SP, but not the cholinergic, component may be reduced by CGRP, suggesting a selective interaction between the two types of neuron containing these peptides [12]. The overall peristaltic reflex can, therefore, be modulated by intrinsic nerves which evoke NANC-mediated responses and which originate from other parts of the gut. The exact anatomical relationships between these neurons and the stimulus which initiates their firing remains obscure.

► The peristaltic wave, enabling the progression of a bolus through the intestine, consists of two reflexes.
► The enteric ascending excitatory reflex causes a contraction in the intestine occurring above the site of bolus stimulation: ACh is the predominant neurotransmitter involved in this reflex, although SP is thought to play a role in maintaining the reflex.
► The enteric descending inhibitory reflex causes a relaxation below the site of stimulation: VIP may be the predominant neurotransmitter involved in this reflex; in addition, VIP antiserum has been shown to enhance the ascending excitatory response.

Involvement in sphincter function

Distension of an area of gut immediately proximal to a sphincter activates descending NANC-mediated inhibitory nerve responses which relax the sphincter muscle. The mechanisms of this reflex are no different from the descending inhibitory reflex of peristalsis (see [1]). However, the identity of the neurotransmitter need not necessarily be the same as that found in other regions of the gut.

Descending excitatory reflexes may also affect sphincter function. For example, oesophageal acidification in cats evokes a SP-dependent reflex which contracts the lower oesophageal sphincter. However, in man it is questionable whether such a reflex exists [13].

Involvement in colonic function

The mechanisms by which non-propulsive contractions are evoked and the means by which the proximal colon can exhibit segmentation (haustral contractions) and anti-peristalsis are poorly understood. Such a pattern of motility is necessary to facilitate fluid and ion absorption, partly by allowing sufficient time for this to occur and partly by mixing of the relatively viscous contents.

Atropine-sensitive mechanisms have been implicated in the segmentation of rabbit colon, whereas atropine-resistant neuronal mechanisms are implicated in anti-peristalsis [14]. However, once sufficient absorption has occurred, it is not clear how the colon can then switch from segmentation and anti-peristalsis to peristalsis, and the nature of the stimulus is unknown. Is there a continuous but slow movement of colonic contents down the intestine, or does the colon 'sense' the need to propel a sufficiently dry faecal mass from the proximal to distal region of the colon? Perhaps endogenous opioids suppress the descending reflex of peristalsis, facilitating non-propulsive intestinal movement; naloxone accelerates colonic transit in normal volunteers [15]. However, if this is the final modulatory pathway, what are the stimuli that control opioid activity?

3. Fluid secretion and absorption

In healthy individuals, neuronal secretomotor reflexes are activated by the mechanical and chemical stimuli that occur during digestion to lubricate and dilute the intraluminal contents, facilitating their transport along the gut. Mechanically induced (normal peristalsis and mixing) secretion may be partly mediated by cholinergic fibres, although a non-cholinergic pathway has also been proposed. For the latter, the strongest neurotransmitter candidates are SP and VIP. As with the peristaltic reflex, their activity and release may also be modulated by somatostatin- and enkephalin-containing neurons [16].

4. Mucus secretion

Mechanical stimulation of the villous cells will release mucus, by non-neuronal mechanisms, to lubricate the passage of food and to protect the underlying epithelial cells from damage. Neuronal modulation has yet to be conclusively demonstrated.

5. Blood flow

In cat ileum, mechanical stimulation releases 5-HT from enterochromaffin cells which, in turn, may directly or indirectly activate VIP-containing neurons and thereby evoke vasodilation (see [17] for references). Similarly, VIP may mediate the colonic and rectal vasodilation evoked by mechanical stimulation of the rectum or by pelvic nerve stimulation. Such reflexes may form part of the larger defaecation reflex (see [18] for references). Blood flow may also be modulated by the chemical composition of the distending bolus (e.g. the presence of bile salts), activating local axon reflexes utilizing VIP-containing neurons.

By means of reflexes such as those described above, changes in intestinal motility and secretion are linked to a co-ordinated change in blood flow. Their close relationship is illustrated by experiments with cat small intestine. Distension evoked an ascending excitatory and a descending inhibitory reflex. Mucosal blood flows above and below the area of distension were also increased, but the magnitude of increase was greater on the anal side. Detectable VIP release was also greater anally than orally [19]. Thus, the maximum increase both in VIP and blood flow occurred in the area of the intestine which had to relax (perhaps also in response to VIP) in order to receive the advancing food bolus. The dilated vasculature promotes an efficient exchange of ions and fluid.

- ▶ Distension of gut immediately proximal to a sphincter activates descending NANC-mediated inhibitory nerve responses which relax the sphincter muscle.
- ▶ The stimuli that control colonic contractions are less well understood.
- ▶ VIP may be the predominant neurotransmitter involved in regulating fluid secretion and blood flow; a maximum increase in both VIP and blood flow occurs in the relaxed intestine below the advancing bolus.

Involvement of NANC systems in the pathophysiology of gut motility disorders

The involvement of neuronal NANC-mediated responses in disorders of gut motility has been described by Furness and Costa [1]. Complex mechanisms may often be involved, with both gut reflexes and gut–spinal cord/brain pathways playing important roles. It should also be remembered that disorders of intestinal fluid secretion and motility often coincide, an essential requirement for washing out bacteria, toxins or parasite invasions from the lumen of the gut.

1. Loss of sphincter function

Abnormalities in oesophageal peristalsis and in lower oesophageal sphincter function occur in diffuse oesophageal spasm. This condition can progress into achalasia, in which oesophageal peristalsis is absent, resting lower oesophageal sphincter pressure is elevated and there is incomplete sphincter relaxation with swallowing. These changes have been attributed mostly to a loss of neuronal, excitatory and inhibitory NANC-mediated responses within the lower oesophageal sphincter [creating an imbalance between the inhibitory and excitatory innervation, so that a descending bolus cannot easily activate a descending inhibitory reflex and open the sphincter (achalasia) and/or a failure of propagation of peristalsis along the oesophagus (diffuse or oesophageal spasm)]. The identities of all of the neurotransmitters involved are not known, but a loss of VIP-containing neurons has been identified in achalasia. Thus, these conditions may be due, at least partly, to a defective descending inhibitory reflex pathway, normally mediated by VIP [11].

Attempts to draw parallel conclusions from the study of VIP fibres in the lower oesophageal sphincter with the aetiology of pyloric stenosis have so far proved inconsistent [11]. However, one study concluded that infantile hypertrophic pyloric stenosis is associated with a loss of peptide immunoreactivity (enkephalin, gastrin-releasing peptide, neuropeptide Y, somatostatin, SP and VIP) in nerve fibres of the circular muscle, but not in the myenteric plexus [20].

2. Gastric stasis

The aetiology of non-ulcer dyspepsia and lower oesophageal reflux is now known, but both conditions are often associated with a reduced gastric motility and rate of emptying. At present, an important means of treatment is the use of the drug metoclopramide. This drug facilitates the release of ACh from gut myenteric neurons, restoring normal gastric motility and co-ordination. The success of metoclopramide led to the development of cisapride and to the identification of renzapride, both of which have a more selective action on gastric cholinergic function, with reduced side-effects [21].

With regard to NANC-mediated mechanisms, the significance of the gut motility stimulants lies in the means by which they increase myenteric cholinergic function. Metoclopramide and renzapride are thought to increase ACh release by activating a pre-junctional 5-HT receptor of the 5-HT_4 type [22]. Whether 5-HT_4 receptors are physiologically activated by 5-HT from 5-hydroxytryptaminergic fibres or from enterochromaffin cells is not yet known. Identification of the source of 5-HT might lead to a greater understanding of the role played by 5-HT in the normal functioning of the stomach and in the mechanisms of gastric stasis.

3. Nausea and vomiting

This is a complex reflex mechanism, only part of which involves the gastro-intestinal tract; gastric relaxation and small intestinal retropulsion. An involvement of NANC-mediated neural inhibitory responses is now well established in the mechanism of gastric relaxation. These fibres are activated by vagal efferents, following an emetic stimulus. However, the gastric relaxation does not in itself cause vomiting. Strong contractions of the diaphragm co-ordinated with intercostal muscle activity are essential. Nevertheless, gastric relaxation may facilitate or cause nausea, particularly in functional gut disorders which might be amenable to treatment with gut motility stimulants [22].

The mechanisms by which small intestinal retropulsion can occur are not fully understood, although non-cholinergic excitatory nerve activity (see section headed 'Ascending excitation and descending inhibition') is involved. Neurons containing 5-HT have been implicated, but the evidence is based on data obtained with non-selective drugs; 5-HT has, however, been strongly linked to the mechanisms of cytotoxic-drug-induced emesis [22].

4. Motility disorders associated with pain and inflammation

Normal gastro-intestinal motility may give rise to pain if the gut mucosa is inflamed or in some way sensitized by non-inflammatory algesic substances (e.g. Irritable Bowel Syndrome). Alternatively, pain can be evoked if the mechanical stimulus is sufficiently prolonged or intense. The pain is poorly localized and can give rise to reflex suppression of gut motility. At least part of this reflex is mediated by sympathetic fibres. However, an unknown degree of influence will also be exerted by antidromic release of peptides such as CGRP from the visceral afferent fibres [23]. In cats, intestinal distension, surgery or peritonitis (serosal inflammation) will activate both spinal adrenergic and vagal gastric inhibitory nerve activity [24]. Such mechanisms contribute to the associated paralytic ileus. With regards to peritonitis, the release of inflammatory mediators causes hyperaemia, increased vascular permeability and increased nociceptor activity, at least partly by activation of nerve fibres using ACh and/or other neurotransmitters [25]. Participation of this pathway in the motility changes associated with peritonitis or inflammatory bowel disease remains speculative. There is, nevertheless, an increase in the VIP content found in resected segments of inflamed bowel from patients with Crohn's disease [11].

5. Constipation

There are many causes of constipation, and treatment is often simple. However, patients with chronic or intractable idiopathic constipation have a disorder in the mechanisms of lower bowel motility, sensitivity, innervation, absorptive function and/or defaecation reflexes. Some will have symptoms of faecal incontinence, at least partly due to a reduced sensitivity of the rectum, failing to detect the presence of a faecal mass and close the anal sphincter [26].

Young women with severe constipation do not respond to laxatives (which can exacerbate symptoms [26]). Apart from surgery, treatment of this form of constipation has, therefore, progressed little from 100 years ago when one clinician recommended that patients roll a cannon ball over their abdomen every day for 5 or 10 minutes. From time to time it was suggested that the cannon ball should also be occasionally raised to a certain height 'and brought down on his belly with some force' [27].

To achieve some progress in the treatment of intractable constipation, it may be necessary to turn towards the study of neurotransmitters other than ACh or NA. Preliminary evidence suggests that the opioid antagonist naloxone might benefit some patients. Thus, naloxone reversed constipation in two patients with this disorder, increased faecal wet weights in geriatric patients and accelerated colonic transit in normal volunteers [15, 28]. One study of colon specimens from patients with chronic constipation revealed no difference in enkephalin content when compared with colons from non-constipated patients [29]. However, enkephalin turnover was not measured. The authors did, nevertheless, report a decreased concentration of VIP. Decreased concentrations of VIP were also detected by Milner et al. [30], who found, in addition, an increase in the 5-HT content. The significance of these findings remains to be determined. However, since enkephalins, VIP and 5-HT are so clearly implicated in the physiology of normal gut function, an imbalance in the turnover of one or more of these substances could disrupt colonic function.

► Neuronal NANC-mediated responses are involved in gut motility disorders.
► Achalasia is thought to be brought about by a defective descending inhibitory reflex pathway, normally mediated by VIP.
► Pain can result from inflamed gut mucosa or a prolonged/intense mechanical stimulus; the afferent nerves may develop a heightened sensitivity due to the release of local mediators (e.g. 5-HT, bradykinin, prostaglandins).
► An imbalance in the turnover of enkephalins, VIP and/or 5-HT could disrupt colonic function, resulting in constipation.

Conclusions

► Many different neurotransmitters exist in the enteric nervous system and we are now beginning to understand their functions, in both the normal and diseased gut.

► The peristaltic reflex relies heavily on ACh and additionally on neurotransmitters other than ACh or NA.

► Ascending excitatory and descending inhibitory responses evoked by radial distension, modulate gut motility, secretion and blood flow.

► In some examples, VIP, SP and/or 5-HT are implicated as neurotransmitters; however, there is also a poorly understood species- and/or regional-dependence on the types of neurotransmitters involved.

► Alternatively, identification of the active neurotransmitter may be complicated in some species by the co-localization and release of different neurotransmitters.

► Future evaluation of the function of NANC-mediated neuronal responses will make great advances when selective receptor antagonists and agonists are available for the many substances proposed as neurotransmitters; for 5-HT, this is currently being achieved, although there is still a long way to go.

References

1. Furness, J. B. and Costa, M. (1987) The Enteric Nervous System, Churchill Livingstone, Edinburgh
2. Furness, J. B., Morris, J. L., Gibbins, I. L. and Costa, M. (1989) Chemical coding of neurons and plurichemical transmission. Annu. Rev. Pharmacol. Toxicol. **29**, 289–306
3. Fox, J. E. T. (1989) Control of gastrointestinal motility by peptides: old peptides new tricks—new peptides old tricks. Gastrointestinal Clinics of North America **18**, 163–177
4. Costa, M., Furness, J. B. and Gibbons, I. L. (1986) Chemical coding of enteric neurons. Brain Res. **68**, 217–239
5. Bornstein, J. C. and Furness, J. B. (1988) Correlated electrophysiological and histochemical studies of submucous neurons and their contribution to understanding enteric neural circuits. J. Aut. Nerv. System **25**, 1–13
6. Szurszewski, J. H. and King, B. F. (1989) Physiology of prevertebral ganglia in mammals with special reference to inferior mesenteric ganglion. In Handbook of Physiology: The Gastrointestinal System, Section 6, Vol 1, Part 1 (Wood, J. D., ed.), pp. 519–592, American Physiological Society, Bethesda, M.D., U.S.A.
7. Furness, J. B. and Costa, M. (1982) Enteric inhibitory nerves and VIP. In Vasoactive Intestinal peptide (Said, S. I., ed.), pp. 391–406, Raven Press, New York
8. Grider, J. R. and Makhlouf, G. M. (1990) Regulation of the peristaltic reflex by peptides of the myenteric plexus. Arch. Int. Pharmacodyn. Ther. **303**, 232–251
9. Lin, J. G., Neya, T. and Nakayama, S. (1989) Myenteric 5-HT-containing neurones activate the descending cholinergic excitatory pathway to the circular muscle of guinea-pig ileum. Br. J. Pharmacol. **98**, 982–988
10. Daniel, E. E. and Kostolanska, F. (1989) Functional studies of nerve projections in the canine intestine. Can. J. Physiol. Pharmacol. **67**, 1074–1085
11. Biancani, P., Beinfeld, M. C., Coy, D. H., Hillemeier, C., Walsh, J. H. and Behar, J. (1988) Dysfunction of the gastrointestinal tract. Vasoactive intestinal peptide in peristalsis and sphincter function. In Vasoactive Intestinal Peptide and Related Peptides (Said, S. I. and Mutt, V., eds.), Ann. N.Y. Acad. Sci. **527**, 546–567
12. Holzer, P., Bartho, L., Matusák, O. and Bauer, V. (1989) Calcitonin gene-related peptide action on intestinal circular muscle. Am. J. Physiol. **256**, G546–G552
13. Vakil, N. B., Kahrilas, P. J., Dodds, W. J. and Vanagunas, A. (1989) Absence of an upper eosophageal sphincter response to acid reflux. Am. J. Gastroenterol. **84**, 606–610
14. Bouvier, M. and Jule, Y. (1983) Intramural neural mechanisms involved in the antiperistaltic and the segmentation movements of the large intestine. In Gastrointestinal Motility (Labo, G. and Bortolotti, M., eds.), pp. 171–172, Coratina International, Verona, Italy
15. Kaufman, P. N., Krevsky, B., Malmud, L. S., Maurer, A. H., Somers, M. B., Siegel, J. A. and Fisher, R. S. (1988) Role of opiate receptors in the regulation of colonic transit. Gastroenterology **94**, 1351–1356
16. Cassuto, J., Jodal, M., Sjövall, H. and Lundgren, O. (1981) Nervous control of intestinal secretion. Clin. Res. Rev. **1** (**Suppl. 1**), 11–21
17. Eklund, S., Fahrnkrug, J., Jodal, M., Lundgren, O., Schaffalitzky de Muckadell, O. B. and Sjöqvist, A. (1980) Vasoactive intestinal polypeptide, 5-hydroxytryptamine and reflex hyperaemia in the small intestine of the cat. J. Physiol. **302**, 549–557
18. Andersson, P.-O., Bloom, S. R., Edwards, A. V., Järhult, J. and Melander, S. (1983) Neural vasodilator control in the rectum of the cat and its mediation by vasoactive intestinal polypeptide. J. Physiol. **344**, 49–67
19. Sjöqvist, A. and Fahrenkrug, J. (1987) Release of vasoactive intestinal polypeptide anally of a local distension of the feline small intestine. Acta Physiol. Scand. **130**, 433–438
20. Wattchow, D. A., Cass, D. T., Furness, J. B., Costa, M., O'Brien, P. E., Little, K. E. and Pitkin, J. (1987) Abnormalities of peptide-containing nerve fibers in infantile hypertrophic pyloric stenosis. Gastroenterology **92**, 443–448
21. Sanger, G. J. and King, F. D. (1988) From metoclopramide to selective gut stimulants and 5-HT_3 receptor antagonists. Drug Des. Delivery **3**, 273–295
22. Sanger, G. J. (1990) New anti-emetic drugs. Can. J. Physiol. Pharmacol. **68**, 314–324
23. Dockray, G. J. and Sharkey, K. A. (1986) Neurochemistry of visceral afferent neurones. In Prog. Brain Res.: Visceral Sensation (Cevero, F. and Morrison, J. F. B., eds.), **67**, 133–148, Elsevier, Amsterdam
24. Abrahamsson, H. (1986) Non-adrenergic, non-cholinergic nervous control of gastrointestinal motility patterns. Arch. Int. Pharmacodyn. Ther. **280** (**Suppl.**), 50–61
25. Brunsson, I., Sjöqvist, A., Jodal, M. and Lundgren, O. (1985) Mechanisms underlying the intestinal fluid secretion evoked by nociceptive serosal stimulation of the rat. Naunyn-Schmiedeberg's Arch. Pharmacol. **328**, 439–445
26. Read, N. W. and Timms, J. M. (1986) Defecation and the pathophysiology of constipation. Clin. Gastroenterol. **15**, 937–965
27. Editorial (1887) Cannon-balls in chronic constipation. Br. Med. J., Nov. 26th, p. 1171
28. Kreek, M. J., Paris, P., Bartol, M. A. and Mueller, D. (1984) Effects of short term oral administration of the specific opioid antagonist naloxone on fecal evacuation in geriatric patients. Gastroenterology **86**, 1144
29. Koch, T. R., Carney, A., Go, L. and Go, V. L. W. (1988) Idiopathic chronic constipation is associated with decreased colonic vasoactive intestinal peptide. Gastroenterology **94**, 300–310
30. Milner, P., Lincoln, J., Crowe, R., Kamm, M., Lennard-Jones, J. E. and Burnstock, G. (1989) Serotonin is increased and VIP decreased in the sigmoid colon in idiopathic constipation. Gut 30, A715

4

The pathophysiology of cystic fibrosis in the airways

Duncan M. Geddes and Eric Alton
Brompton Hospital, Fulham Road, London SW3 6HP, U.K.

Introduction

Cystic fibrosis (CF) is an inherited disorder which is expressed most strikingly at three different sites: the airways, the gastro-intestinal tract and the sweat glands. The clinical consequences are, at first sight, very different with bacterial infection in the lungs leading to respiratory failure, pancreatic insufficiency predisposing to malnutrition, and high concentrations of electrolytes (chiefly sodium and chloride) in the sweat causing little disease, but providing a convenient measurement for diagnosis. Since the disorder is caused by a defect in a single gene, the same defect must be responsible for the changes in three different organ systems. This defect appears to be one of epithelial cell membrane transport. In particular, alterations in chloride transport are central to the pathophysiology of CF, although changes in sodium and water transport are also likely to be important. Furthermore, the recent identification of the defective gene on chromosome 7 has led to a prediction of the structure and probable function of the affected protein. The structure is that of a transmembrane protein which resembles P-glycoprotein, thought to cause multiple drug resistance in cancer cells by exporting a variety of molecules including cations, peptides and ionophores [1]. The protein may, therefore, have a wider role in regulating transmembrane transport and has thus been labelled CF transmembrane conductance regulator (CFTR).

This chapter attempts to relate the altered physiology of CF airways to the pulmonary disease and, in particular, to explore the link between epithelial ion transport and bacterial colonization, infection and subsequent lung damage.

Normal lung defences

Normal lung defences may be considered under two headings: mechanical and immune. The mechanical defences are involved in keeping the lung sterile by preventing bacterial access and by rapidly clearing any bacteria that enter. These systems operate predominantly in the conducting airways. Immune mechanisms are a second line of defence which operate once micro-organisms have entered the airways and set up residence. These are particularly important in the alveoli where mechanical clearance systems are very slow and inefficient, although immune-mediated inflammation also becomes important in the conducting airways when these become colonized, and may play a role in preventing such colonization.

Mechanical clearance

Inhaled and aspirated particles that penetrate beyond the larynx may be treated in one of three ways: large particles (>10 μm) impact onto the surface of the central airways to be rapidly cleared by coughing or mucociliary transport; small particles (<2 μm) remain suspended in the inspired air and are breathed out with the next expired air; and intermediate-sized particles are deposited in the small airways and alveoli and are subsequently cleared by mucociliary transport (small airways) or a combination of phagocytosis and lymphatic drainage (alveoli). In CF, cough and alveolar clearance mechanisms are normal, at least until secondarily altered by infective lung damage; thus, the mechanism most directly affected by this condition is mucociliary clearance.

The airway epithelial surface is composed chiefly of ciliated columnar cells with a few mucus-secreting goblet cells. Between this surface layer and the cartilage of the large airways are the mucus glands. The surface is covered by a layer of airway-surface liquid (ASL) which is propelled by the cilia from the periphery towards the larynx for eventual swallowing or expectoration. The surface layer is complex and best considered as composed of a surface gel, derived from the goblet cells and mucus glands, which lies on top of a sol layer derived from the remainder of the airway epithelium. The volume, composition and regulation of this sol layer have been studied in little depth, but these properties of ASL are central to an understanding of CF. As the airway secretions move centrally from the peripheral airways, the surface area of the airways progressively diminishes and consequently the ASL layer must either become thicker, move faster or be removed as it reaches the central airways. There is some evidence to suggest that transport is faster in the trachea than in the bronchi, but it is likely that evaporation and absorption also contribute. Evaporation is important for cooling in dogs but not in man, and the processes of transepithelial secretion and absorption need, therefore, to be finely balanced at all airway levels. Secretion presumably dominates at the periphery while absorption dominates centrally.

Transport of ions and water

The mechanisms involved in transepithelial secretion and absorption involve the transport of ions and water [2]. Most data have come from dogs, studies on human airways being few and incomplete. The most important ions are sodium and chloride, with chloride movement into the lumen responsible for secretion and sodium transport responsible for absorption. The ubiquitous Na^+,K^+-ATPase, situated on the serosal surface of the airway epithelial cells, is responsible for maintaining low intracellular concentrations of sodium. This is an active energy-requiring process and can be inhibited by ouabain. In tissues in which sodium absorption dominates (Fig. 1), sodium moves into the cell from the mucosal surface

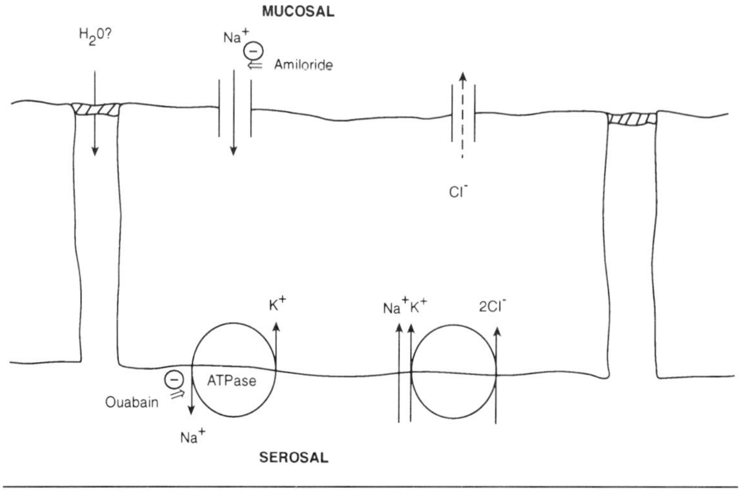

Fig. 1. Principal suggested ion movements across Na^+-absorbing epithelia

Chloride secretion represents only a small portion of the total current, the principal ion moved being Na^+, absorbed through mucosally sited channels. Both Na^+ and Cl^- are accompanied by the opposite ion to maintain electrical neutrality. These movements are not shown on the diagram for simplicity. Amiloride and ouabain inhibit ion-transport at the sites shown.

through specific channels down this favourable gradient created by the ATPase. This is a purely passive process and can be blocked by the specific sodium channel blocker amiloride. Water osmotically follows this net ion movement, probably through paracellular pathways. If chloride secretion predominates (Fig. 2), the same gradient for sodium entry into the cell is used to move sodium through the serosal surface. Again this is a passive process energized by the ATPase activity. This sodium movement is coupled to the entry of both chloride and potassium through the serosally sited $Na^+/2Cl^-/K^+$ co-transporter, which can be inhibited by 'loop' diuretics such as frusemide and bumetanide. Chloride is now accumulated within the cell, and is moved out through the mucosal cell surface down a favourable electrochemical gradient. Again this is purely a passive process occurring through specific chloride channels, and again water follows osmotically through paracellular pathways.

A number of controlling mechanisms for chloride secretion have been observed. For instance, activation of any of the three known second messenger pathways increases chloride secretion. Thus, for example, adrenoceptor agonists acting via cyclic AMP, bradykinin via increasing intracellular free calcium, or phorbol esters via activation of protein kinase C, all stimulate chloride transport. It is likely that each of the second messengers acts directly on chloride channels to increase their probability of being open (Fig. 3). The control of sodium absorption is much less well understood, apart from its known dependence on Na^+,K^+-ATPase and its inhibition by amiloride.

The above noted agents have been useful in studies exploring the control of electrolyte and water transport across the respiratory epithelium, but the balance of physiological influences and, in particular, the local stimuli that ensure the fine control of ASL are still far from understood.

The rate of transport of ASL is dependent on ciliary beat frequency as well as on the viscoelastic properties of the overlying mucus. The cilia beat at 10–14 Hz and this intrinsic frequency appears to be relatively constant at

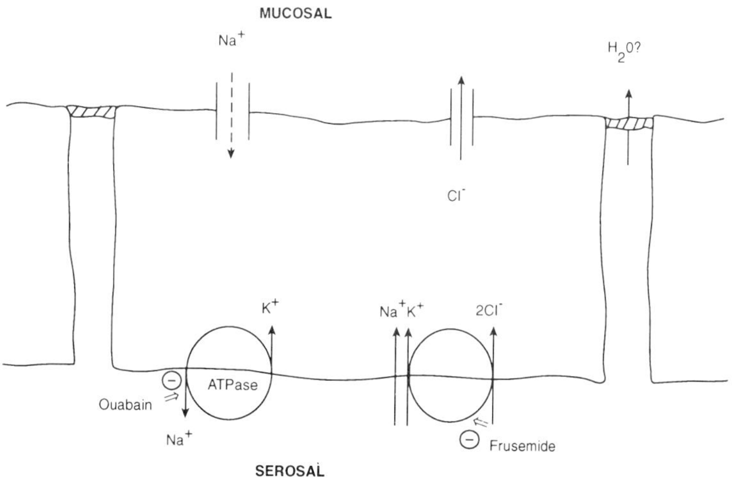

Fig. 2. Principal suggested ion movements across the canine trachea
Mucosal sodium entry represents only a small proportion of the total current. Ouabain and frusemide inhibit ion transport at the sites shown.

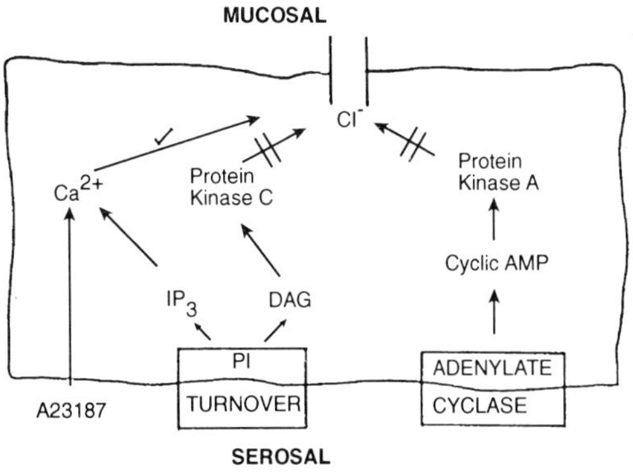

Fig. 3. Schematic representation of second messenger pathways interacting with mucosal airway epithelial chloride channels

In CF activation can occur via Ca^{2+}, but not by protein kinase A or C. Abbreviations used: DAG, diacylglycerol; IP_3, inositol triphosphate; PI, phosphoinositide. A23187 is a Ca^{2+}-ionophore promoting Ca^{2+} entry into the cell.

different airway levels and under varying conditions of temperature and humidity. However, both ciliary function and mucus visco-elasticity are easily impaired by disease (see below).

Cellular and immune defences

Pulmonary cellular immune defences are particularly important at the alveolar level where phagocytic macrophages are constantly 'on patrol'. These macrophages release chemotactic factors when activated and so promote inflammation and immune activity when micro-organisms reach the alveoli. In the airways, the number of phagocytic cells is small under normal circumstances, but a variety of proteins in ASL help to inhibit bacterial attachment and growth. These include ferritin and lysozyme, and some components of the complement system, as well as locally produced immunoglobulin A (IgA) and perhaps some serum-derived IgG. Since there is no evidence that any of these cellular or immune defences are impaired by the genetic abnormality in CF they will not be discussed further.

Bacterial adherence

The airways are normally sterile and, although bacteria are repeatedly aspirated and inhaled, they are rapidly removed. Adherence of bacteria to the epithelium appears to be an important first step in colonization of the lower respiratory tract which precedes multiplication. Undoubtedly, the main defences against such adherence are the ASL and mucociliary clearance; however, other factors also appear to be important. Adherence requires an interaction between cell surface receptors and bacterial surface polysaccharides (adhesins); these receptors are normally masked by surface fibronectin and only exposed when this is removed by airway proteases. The receptors themselves have not been fully characterized but surface glycolipids containing *N*-acetylneuraminic acid or *N*-acetylglucosamine are likely to be involved in adherence of the bacterium *Pseudomonas aeruginosa*. Bacteria may also adhere to amino sugars in the mucus layer, although such adherence is much less likely to lead to permanent colonization. The epithelial surface pH appears to be an important defence against adherence, as does the surface charge, and these factors may be particularly important in CF. The respiratory epithelium is negatively charged relative to the subcutaneous space by approximately −20 mV in the trachea falling to −10 mV in segmental bronchi, the potential difference approaching zero peripherally. Clearly such a surface charge is likely to result in an alteration in mucus and cell-surface chemistry and may therefore be an important defence against bacterial adherence.

► Normal lung defences involve mechanisms for preventing bacterial adherence to and colonization of the airways; the main defences against adherence are the ASL and mucociliary clearance, the latter mechanism being most greatly disrupted in cystic fibrosis.
► Secretion and absorption across the airway epithelial surface involve the transport of ions and water: the movement of Cl^- into the lumen is responsible for secretion, while Na^+ transport is involved in absorption processes.
► Secretion of Cl^- is activated by second messenger pathways and inhibited by frusemide; Na^+ absorption is dependent on Na^+,K^+-ATPase and is inhibited by amiloride.

Abnormalities in cystic fibrosis

It has long been recognized that CF patients characteristically demonstrate viscous secretions within the affected organs. In the airways these secretions are commonly infected with *Staphylococcus aureus* and *P. aeruginosa*, leading to much of the morbidity and mortality associated with the disease. In attempting to dissect the aetiology of these abnormalities, studies have focused on the various aspects which should normally enable the airways to be cleared.

Cilia appear to have normal ultrastructure in CF, although products of *P. aeruginosa* are able to induce malformations. These observations exemplify the problems encountered in many of these studies, that is the ability to distinguish between the primary genetic abnormality and the secondary effects of bacterial infection. The overlying sol phase of the airway secretions is difficult to assess directly. However, it is likely that the principal effect of the genetic abnormality is targeted at this point. As explained more fully in the next section the ion transport abnormalities in CF make it likely that the sol layer will be relatively dehydrated in these patients. An *in vivo* study which measured the water vapour partial pressure of inspired air at the pharynx showed no differences between normal and CF subjects when inhaling ambient air [3]. However, when the air temperature was raised to 48°C, CF patients showed a significantly reduced partial pressure suggesting that, when evaporation is increased, CF upper airways cannot produce sufficient water. Since the sol volume is likely to critically influence the efficacy of ciliary beating, an abnormality of ion and hence water transport may be expected to produce many of the observed abnormalities in CF.

The gel layer/mucus in CF has been shown to be abnormal in several respects. The glycoprotein component is altered in composition as well as being increased in quantity. The mucus also shows a decreased water content [4] consistent with similar findings in secretions from the pancreas, gastro-intestinal and reproductive tracts. This reduced hydration may once again link with the abnormal ion and water transport described above.

A further recently described abnormality of CF mucus is the oversulphation of high-molecular-weight glycoconjugates [5] which are secreted into the airways as part of the mucosal defence mechanism. These macromolecules are packaged with sulphate in vesicles within the Golgi apparatus prior to release into the airways. Since the sulphate ions are transported across the cell membranes, a defect of anion transport more widespread than just that of Cl^- is indicated by this study. It is suggested that the oversulphation may alter not only the properties of the secreted mucus, but also the interaction between bacteria and the macromolecules on the airway surface, perhaps favouring colonization. Thus, again, changes in ion transport may link to much of the observed pathology in the airways in CF.

The ion transport defects *per se* have several characteristic manifestations in the patient *in vivo*. As described in the next section the chloride impermeability of the sweat duct epithelium leads to the characteristically raised Na^+ and Cl^- concentrations in sweat from these patients. This abnormality also leads to an elevated (more negative) potential difference (PD) across the ductal epithelium. By inserting an electrode into a sweat droplet emerging from the duct, and comparing this with an electrode placed in contact with interstitial fluid, Quinton and Bijman [6] demonstrated that the mean PD of CF patients is approximately twice normal.

These observations are consistent with findings in the lungs; Knowles et al. [7] showed a similarly elevated PD in CF airways and, since this increased PD is retained in cell culture free from infection, it is likely that this abnormality is related to the genetic defect, rather than to a secondary effect of infection or a circulating factor. This elevated PD may be useful as an adjunct to diagnosis in CF patients [8].

Causes of abnormalities

An abnormality of the transport of Na^+ and/or Cl^- within sweat glands is the explanation for the high electrolyte concentrations in CF sweat. In 1983 Quinton [9] evaluated this abnormality by demonstrating that, in the isolated sweat duct *in vitro*, the epithelial cells lining the duct are impermeable to chloride ions. Normally, Na^+ is actively reabsorbed from the lumen of the duct moving down an electrochemical gradient created by the ubiquitous Na^+,K^+-ATPase, with Cl^- following passively. Because of the Cl^- impermeability in CF, the apical membrane is markedly depolarized compared with normal, thus reducing the driving force for Na^+ entry. Therefore, both Na^+ and Cl^- are prevented from being reabsorbed, in turn leading to the increase in electrolyte concentrations on the skin surface. Because of the Cl^- transport abnormalities the ductal epithelial cells have a much larger (more negative) PD across their surfaces.

Parallel studies in the airways were first reported by Knowles et al. [7] when they demonstrated that both nasal and lower airway epithelia also have a more negative PD across their surfaces. However, the cause of this abnormality appears to be more complex than in the sweat duct. Chloride impermeability is certainly present and has been demonstrated both *in vivo* and *in vitro*. In normal subjects, superfusion *in vivo* of the nasal mucosa with a solution containing low Cl^- concentrations induces a movement of Cl^- into the airway lumen, thereby rendering the PD more negative. In patients with CF this change is absent, suggesting Cl^- impermeability [7]. *In vitro*, nasal polyps obtained from CF and non-CF patients have been mounted in Ussing chambers to measure their bioelectric characteristics (see also Chapter 5) [10, 11]. When radiolabelled Na^+ and Cl^- were added to the chambers, a reduced movement of Cl^- across the epithelium was demonstrated, as well as the expected larger PD. However, these experiments also showed that Na^+ absorption from the mucosal surface was markedly increased in CF. Further evidence for this abnormality comes from the *in vivo* application to the airway surface of amiloride, which inhibits Na^+ absorption. In normal subjects amiloride reduces PD by between 45 and 65%, whereas in CF patients this fall was approximately 90% [7]. In addition, because Na^+ absorption is dependent on Na^+,K^+-ATPase function, it would be predicted that the rate of pumping might in turn be increased in CF. In agreement with this is the finding that the ouabain-sensitive component of oxygen consumption in airway cells is significantly greater in CF [12]. Finally, recent intracellular microelectrode studies suggest that it is the increased sodium absorption that is principally responsible for the raised PD in the airways, which is in marked contrast to the situation seen in the sweat gland duct [13].

The molecular basis of these changes in ion transport has been elegantly elucidated. The patch-clamp technique allows single ionic channels to be studied under voltage clamp conditions. A number of studies have now demonstrated that, in non-CF airways when a channel is studied in the cell-attached configuration (in its normal position in the cell membrane), Cl^- channels can be identified following application of any agent that raises cellular cyclic AMP levels [14, 15]. In contrast, in CF cells, channels are never seen following this type of stimulation [15, 16]. However, if the patch of membrane containing the channel is now excised, channel activity is stimulated both in CF and non-CF cells. Therefore, it is an abnormality of Cl^- channel control, rather than the absence of channels, which appears to underlie the CF defect. Cyclic AMP activates protein kinase A within cells and this enzyme then phosphorylates various effector proteins. Addition of the catalytic subunit of protein kinase A also fails to activate CF Cl^- channels indicating a defect downstream of cyclic AMP production in these cells [17, 18]. Furthermore, activation by protein kinase C is also defective in CF, suggesting a generalized defect of protein phosphorylation by these kinases [19, 20]. The Cl^- channel, however, can be normally activated in CF by agents elevating free intracellular Ca^{2+} [21] (Fig. 3). Thus, either more than one type of Cl^- channel exists, for which there is increasing evidence, or the second messenger pathway acts on different cellular substrates in channel regulation. Sodium channels have proved more difficult to study as their conductance is much smaller and their occurrence is less frequent. However, preliminary studies [22] suggest their regulation is also defective, which is in keeping with the *in vivo* and *in vitro* experiments described above. That the genetic abnormality on chromosome 7 is indeed linked to Cl^- impermeability has been shown recently by an elegant study involving the introduction of normal DNA coding for CFTR into CF airway cells, thereby reversing the abnormal Cl^- transport present in these cells [23, 24].

Since the identification of the CF gene [25], the CFTR has been identified and purified [26] and further aspects of the control of the Cl^- channel have been studied [27, 28].

▶ CF patients exhibit bacterially infected viscous secretions within the affected organs.
▶ The overlying sol layer of the airway epithelial surface in CF is dehydrated as a result of ion transport abnormalities.
▶ Mucus within the airways of CF patients contains oversulphated high-molecular-weight glycoconjugates which are thought to favour bacterial colonization.
▶ Epithelial cells of sweat gland ducts and of the airways are impermeable to Cl^- in CF; these changes in ion transport appear to be caused by an abnormality of ion channel control, rather than an absence of channels.

Cystic fibrosis and lung damage

From the above discussion it can be concluded that, in the airways, the likely consequence of both patterns of ion transport abnormalities is a reduction in the water content of ASL. Increased Na^+ absorption will favour dehydration of the sol layer, and lack of Cl^- secretion will prevent the rehydration 'fine tuning' that is likely to be present normally. As mucociliary clearance depends upon a critical sol volume for normal ciliary activity, these ionic changes are likely to underlie the impaired clearances seen in these patients.

From the cystic fibrosis defect to lung damage

The ion transport abnormalities associated with CF form the first link in the chain of events which leads to lung damage. This damage develops slowly and can be considered in two stages. The first stage is bacterial colonization of the airways which is not in itself damaging, and the second is bacterial multiplication which, by inducing a local inflammatory response, injures the airways and sets up vicious cycles of progressive lung damage.

The link between altered ion transport and bacterial colonization is not yet clear. Bacterial adherence mechanisms are likely to be altered by the change in surface charge or the altered sulphation of glycoproteins, but there is no direct evidence to support this. A second possibility is an alteration in mucus glyoproteins leading to suboptimal airway defence or clearance. Mucus is difficult to collect and study in the crucial presymptomatic stage of CF lung disease and so evidence is again lacking, and by the time frank lung disease has developed, any effects of the ionic abnormality on mucus are overshadowed by the products of infection and inflammation. The factor most likely to induce colonization is the effect that CF has on the sol layer of ASL, and the consequent changes in mucociliary clearance. Strong support for the importance of this factor is that nebulized amiloride improves mucociliary clearance in CF [29].

The second stage in the development of CF lung damage is more closely linked to bacterial products and host inflammation than to the ion transport abnormality. The importance of these secondary mechanisms is best illustrated by considering the dramatic improvement in treatments for CF lung disease over the past 30 years. Previously, severe lung damage occurred in early childhood and survival into adult life was rare. Nowadays, survival with relatively good lung function into adult life is usual and the prognosis is improving. These changes have taken place while the ion transport defect remained unaltered and are probably due to improved anti-microbial therapy and a greater awareness of the need for good nutrition.

The ways in which infection and inflammation continue to cause lung damage are complex and involve a number of tissue-damaging factors such as protease derived both from bacteria and neutrophils. Vicious cycles then develop in which airway damage as well as bacterial and immune cell products further impair lung clearance mechanisms. This in turn encourages bacterial growth and increased inflammation which leads on to further damage. The details of these processes are beyond the scope of this chapter.

▶ The ion transport abnormalities of CF result, ultimately, in lung damage; this damage can be considered in two stages—bacterial colonization and bacterial multiplication.
▶ As effective mucociliary clearance depends upon a critical sol volume, the most likely cause of bacterial colonization is the dehydration of this layer caused by abnormal ion transport.

▶ Bacterial multiplication induces a local inflammatory response, injures the airways and sets up vicious cycles of progressive lung damage.

References

1. Endicott, J. A. and Ling, V. (1989) The biochemistry of P-glycoprotein-mediated multidrug resistance. Annu. Rev. Biochem. **58**, 137–171
2. Welsh, M. J. (1987) Electrolyte transport by airway epithelia. Physiol. Rev. **67**, 1143–1184
3. Primiano, F. P., Saidel, G. M., Montague, F. W., Kruse, K. L., Green, C. G. and Horowitz, J. G. (1988) Water vapour and temperature dynamics in the upper airways of normal and CF subjects. Eur. Respir. J. **1**, 407–414
4. Matthews, L. W., Spector, S., Lemm, J. and Potter, J. L. (1963) Studies of pulmonary secretions from patients with cystic fibrosis, bronchiectasis and laryngectomy. Am. Rev. Respir. Dis. **88**, 199–204
5. Cheng, P. W., Boat, T. F., Cranfill, K., Yankaskas, J. R. and Boucher, R. C. (1989) Increased sulfation of glycoconjugates by cultured nasal epithelial cells from patients with cystic fibrosis. J. Clin. Invest. **84**, 68–72
6. Quinton, P. M. and Bijman, J. (1983) Higher bioelectric potentials due to decreased chloride absorption in the sweat glands of patients with cystic fibrosis. N. Engl. J. Med. **308**, 1185–1189
7. Knowles, M., Gatzy, J. and Boucher, R. Z. (1981) Increased bioelectric potential difference across respiratory epithelia in cystic fibrosis. N. Engl. J. Med. **305**, 1489–1495
8. Alton, E. W. F. W., Currie, D., Logan-Sinclair, R., Warner, J. O., Hodson, M. E. and Geddes, D. M. (1990) Nasal potential difference: a clinical diagnostic test for cystic fibrosis. Eur. Respir. J. **3**, 922–926
9. Quinton, P. M. (1983) Chloride impermeability in cystic fibrosis. Nature (London) **301**, 421–422
10. Knowles, M., Gatzy, J. and Boucher, R. (1983) Relative ion permeabilities of normal and cystic fibrosis nasal epithelium. J. Clin. Invest. **71**, 1410–1417
11. Knowles, M. R., Stutts, M. J., Spock, A., Fischer, N., Gatzy, J. T. and Boucher, R. C. (1983) Abnormal ion permeation through cystic fibrosis respiratory epithelium. Science **221**, 1067–1070
12 Stutts, M. J., Knowles, M. R., Gatzy, J. T. and Boucher, R. C. (1986) Oxygen consumption and ouabain binding sites in cystic fibrosis nasal epithelium. Paediatr. Res. **20**, 1316–1320
13. Willumsen, N. J., Davis, C. W. and Boucher, R. C. (1989) Cellular Cl^- transport in cultured cystic fibrosis airway epithelium. Am. J. Physiol. **256**, C1045–C1053
14. Welsh, M. J. (1986) An apical-membrane chloride channel in human tracheal epithelium. Science **232**, 1648–1650
15. Frizzell, R. A., Rechkemmer, G. and Shoemaker, R. L. (1986) Altered regulation of airway epithelial cell chloride in cystic fibrosis. Science **233**, 558–560
16. Welsh, M. J. and Liedtke, C. M. (1986) Chloride and potassium channels in cystic fibrosis epithelia. Nature (London) **322**, 467–470
17. Li, M., McCann, J. D., Liedtke, C. M., Nairn, A. C., Greengard, P. and Welsh, M. J. (1988) Cyclic AMP-dependent protein kinase opens chloride channels in normal but not cystic fibrosis airway epithelium. Nature (London) **331**, 358–360
18. Schoumacher, R. A., Shoemaker, R. L., Halm, D. R., Tallant, E. A., Wallace, R. W. and Frizzell, R. A. (1987) Phosphorylation fails to activate chloride channels for cystic fibrosis airway cells. Nature (London) **330**, 752–754
19. Hwang, T.-C., Lu, L., Zeitlin, P. L., Gruenert, D. C., Huganir, R. and Guggino, W. B. (1989) Cl^- channels in CF: lack of activation by protein kinase C and cAMP-dependent protein kinase. Science **244**, 1351–1353
20. Li, M., McCann, J. D., Anderson, M. P., Clancy, J. P., Liedtke, C., Nairn, A. C., Greengard, P. and Welsh, M. J. (1989) Regulation of chloride channels by protein kinase C in normal and cystic fibrosis airway epithelia. Science **244**, 1353–1356
21. Boucher, R. C., Cheng, E. H., Paradiso, A. M., Stutts, M. J., Knowles, M. R. and Earp, H. S. (1989) Chloride secretory response of cystic fibrosis human airway epithelia. Preservation of calcium but not protein kinase C- and A-dependent mechanisms. J. Clin. Invest. **84**, 1424–1431
22. Chinet, T., Fullton, J., Boucher, R. and Stutts, J. (1990) Sodium channels in the apical membrane of normal and CF nasal epithelial cells. Paediatr. Pulmonology Suppl. **5**, 209
23. Rich, D. P., Anderson, M. P., Gregory R. J., et al. (1990) Expression of cystic fibrosis transmembrane conductance regulator corrects defective chloride channel regulation in cystic fibrosis airway epithelial cells. Nature (London) **347**, 358–363
24. Drumm, M. L., Pope, H. A., Cliff, W. H., Rommens, J. W., Marvin, S. A., Tsui, L.-C., Collins, F. S., Frizzell, R. A. and Wilson, J. M. (1990) Correction of the cystic fibrosis defect *in vitro* by retrovirus mediated gene transfer. Cell **62**, 1227–1233
25. Rirodan, J. R., Rommens, J. M., Kerem, B., Alon, N., Rozmabel, R., Grzelczak, Z., Zielinski, J., Lok, S., Plavsik, N. and Chon, J. L. (1989) Identification of the cystic fibrosis gene: cloning and characterization of complementary DNA. Science **245**, 1066–1073
26. Berger, H. A., Anderson, M. P., Gregory, R. J., Thompson, S., Howard, P. W., Maurer, R. A., Mulligan, R., Smith, A. E. and Welsh, M. J. (1991) Identification and regulation of the cystic fibrosis transmembrane conductance regulator-generated chloride channel. J. Clin. Invest. **88**, 1422–1431
27. Anderson, M. P., Berger, H. A., Rich, D. P., Gregory, R. J., Smith, A. E. and Welsh, M. J. (1991) Nucleoside triphosphates are required to open the CFTR chloride channel. Cell **67**, 775–784
28. Anderson, M. P. and Welsh, M. J. (1991) Calcium and cAMP activate different chloride channels in the apical membrane of cystic fibrosis epithelia. Proc. Natl Acad. Sci. U.S.A. **88**, 6003–6007
29. App, E. M., King, M., Helfesrieder, R., Kohler, D. and Matthys, H. (1990) Acute and long-term amiloride inhalation in cystic fibrosis lung amerase. A rational approach to cystic fibrosis therapy. Respir. Dis. **141**, 605–612

5

The pathophysiology of cystic fibrosis in the gastro-intestinal tract

J. Hardcastle, P. T. Hardcastle and C. J. Taylor*
Departments of Biomedical Science and Paediatrics*, Sheffield University, Western Bank, Sheffield S10 2TN, U.K.

Introduction

Cystic fibrosis (CF) is the most common lethal genetic defect to affect Caucasian children. One in 2000 babies is born with the disease and at least one in 20 healthy adults carries the gene. The disease affects primarily the respiratory and digestive systems. Recurrent endobronchial infections cause progressive destruction of the lung tissue, while pancreatic exocrine failure leads to malabsorption of nutrients, chronic diarrhoea and weight loss. Afflicted individuals suffer a drastically reduced quality of life with a shortened lifespan and, as a consequence, a great deal of research effort has been directed towards identifying the underlying cause of the disease.

The first clue to the nature of the disease came in 1948 during a heat-wave. Scwachman, a New York paediatrician, noticed that many children admitted to hospital with heat prostration due to excessive sweating suffered from CF. Analysis of the sweat revealed abnormally high levels of sodium and chloride, and this has now become the basis of the 'sweat test' that is used to confirm diagnosis of the disease. The increased sodium and chloride concentrations in the sweat suggest that a disorder of ion transport may be involved in the aetiology of the disease.

Gastro-intestinal effects of cystic fibrosis

Gastro-intestinal dysfunction is a common feature of CF and may indeed be the earliest sign of the disease (Table 1). Up to 15% of patients will present within the first few days of life with meconium ileus, an obstruction of the small intestine by sticky, thick meconium (a mass of desquamated cells, mucus and bile that accumulates in foetal bowel and which is normally discharged shortly after birth). The involvement of the pancreatic and biliary systems explains the deficiency in the luminal phase of digestion in CF. The primary pancreatic abnormality is a reduction in bicarbonate-dependent ductular secretion of water. This leads to dilatation of the ducts with inspissated (thickened) secretions from the enzyme-secreting acini. Severe pancreatic fibrosis and degeneration of the acinar cells are secondary to this process. Thus, the malabsorption in CF results from three separate, but interdependent processes:

— the primary defect in ductular water and bicarbonate secretion
— the reduction in enzyme secretion due to acinar cell destruction
— an inactivation of secreted enzyme by hyperacidity in the upper intestine, secondary to the failure of neutralization of gastric acid by bicarbonate.

The acinar destruction, which also occurs in foetal life, leads to the release of the pancreatic enzyme trypsin into the circulation where it can be detected by sensitive immunoreactive assays which form the basis of a postnatal screening test for the disease.

It is clear, however, that these defects in luminal digestion are not entirely responsible for the intestinal symptoms observed in CF since other pancreatic malformations associated with loss of pancreatic enzymes during foetal life are not accompanied by meconium ileus. Additional factors such as an abnormality in the transport function of the gut may contribute to the intestinal obstruction and abnormal mucous secretion observed in the disorder.

Similar obstructive changes occur in the liver with small bile ducts blocked by inspissated eosinophilic material resembling

Table 1 **Gastro-intestinal manifestations of cystic fibrosis. The symptoms associated with each organ and their frequency of occurrence are indicated**

Organ	Complication	Frequency (%)
Pancreas	Total achylia	85–90
	Abnormal glucose tolerance	15–20
	Diabetes	1–2
Liver	Fatty liver	15–30
	Focal biliary cirrhosis	25
	+ portal hypertension	2–5
Biliary tract	Gallstones	4–12
	Biliary tract obstruction	96
Intestine	Meconium ileus	10–15
	Distal intestinal obstruction syndrome	10–20
	Rectal prolapse	20
	Intussuception	1–5

that found in the pancreatic ducts and acini. The resulting fibrosis from this obstruction is termed 'focal biliary fibrosis' and is characteristic of CF. In time, focal lesions may coalesce and progress to destruction of the liver cells (the hepatocytes); such a condition is known as multilobular biliary cirrhosis. These obstructive changes lead to 'back-pressure' effects such as dilatation of oesophageal veins (varices) and enlargement of the spleen.

▶ The presence of abnormally high levels of sodium and potassium in the sweat forms the basis of the 'sweat test' that is used to confirm diagnosis of CF.
▶ One of the earliest signs of the disease is meconium ileus in newborn babies.
▶ Acinar cell destruction in foetal life leads to release of the pancreatic enzyme, trypsin, into the circulation; the detection of the enzyme by sensitive immunoreactive assays forms the basis of a post-natal screening test for the disease.

Intestinal transport in cystic fibrosis

The gastro-intestinal tract is lined with an epithelium whose cells, the enterocytes, possess a variety of transport processes. These cells are responsible for the movement of ions, nutrients and fluid across the wall of the intestine, and a change in the function of this epithelium could contribute to the intestinal effects of CF described above. Since many intestinal transport mechanisms are electrogenic, one way in which their function can be monitored is by the measurement of transintestinal electrical activity and this can be determined both *in vivo* and in isolated intestinal preparations. However, a major problem in the investigation of intestinal function in human disease is the limited availability of tissue. The recent development of a modification of the Ussing chamber technique to allow the transintestinal electrical activity of intestinal biopsy samples to be measured has extended the range of tissues available for study and provided important information about the transport behaviour of the enterocytes in CF. This approach has been adopted to investigate ion and nutrient transport across jejunal biopsies from children with CF and to compare the behaviour of these tissues with those from a control population.

Measurement of transport in jejunal biopsies

Transintestinal electrical activity can be monitored by mounting the jejunal biopsy sample as a sheet in a modified Ussing chamber

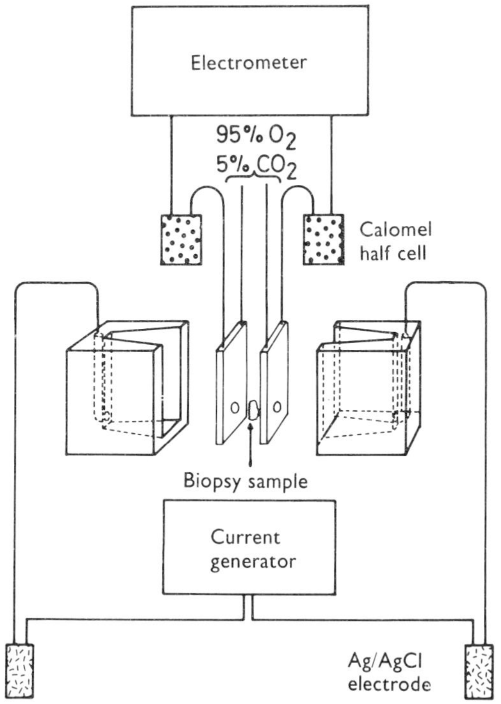

Fig. 1. Modified Ussing chamber for the measurement of transintestinal electrical activity of biopsy samples
The PD is monitored by salt bridge (3% agar in 1 M KCl) electrodes connected via calomel half cells to a differential input electrometer. Current is applied across the tissue by Ag/AgCl electrodes which make contact with mucosal and serosal solutions via wide-bore salt bridges. Tissue resistance is determined from the PD change induced by a 10 μA current pulse and correcting for the resistance of the bathing fluid (Krebs bicarbonate saline). The SCC is calculated from PD and resistance using Ohm's law.

(Fig. 1). The potential difference (PD) across the tissue can then be measured by salt bridge electrodes connected via calomel half cells to a differential input electrometer. The intestine acts as an ohmic resistor and, hence, a change in PD can result from an alteration in the current generated by the tissue, a reflection of net electrogenic ion transport, or from a change in tissue resistance, a measure of passive ionic permeability. Thus, in addition to the PD, tissue resistance is also determined from the PD change induced by applying an external current across the tissue and correcting for the resistance of the bathing medium. From the PD and resistance values, the current generated by the tissue — the short-circuit current (SCC; an index of net electrogenic ion transport) — can be calculated.

All data reported in this chapter are expressed as mean values ±1 standard error of the mean of the number of observations indicated.

Basal electrical activity

Basal electrical activity in the control biopsies (Fig. 2) is very similar to that reported for larger sheets of human intestine [1]. The CF biopsies have a comparable tissue resistance, but the PD and SCC values are significantly lower (Fig. 2).

Electrogenic chloride secretion

Activation of electrogenic ion transport mechanisms generates changes in SCC which can be used to assess the performance of such processes under various conditions. One such mechanism is responsible for the net secretion of chloride ions by the enterocyte [2] and its mode of operation is shown in Fig. 3. Chloride ions are taken up by the enterocyte across its basolateral border by the action of the Na–K–Cl_2 co-transport mechanism, while the sodium that enters the cell is extruded by the sodium pump. Using energy from the sodium gradient, the cell accumulates chloride against its electrochemical potential and so is primed for secretion. When it is stimulated, chloride channels in the luminal membrane open, allowing the accumulated chloride ions to diffuse out into the lumen. Since this process is electrogenic, it depolarizes the luminal membrane, thus reducing the driving force for continued chloride efflux. To prevent attenuation of the secretory process, secretory stimulants activate a second set of ion channels, in this case for potassium, at the basolateral membrane. The resulting potassium efflux causes a hyperpolarization which acts via the low-resistance paracellular pathway between the cells to maintain the luminal membrane potential and hence the driving force for chloride exit. This chloride secretory process in the intestine is very similar to the one that exists in the normal airway

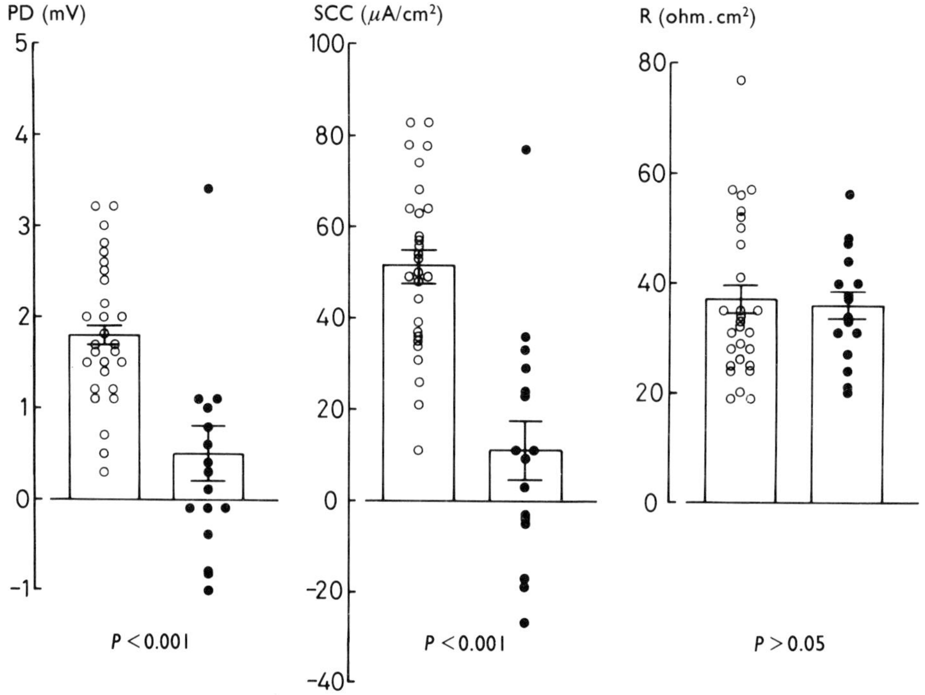

Fig. 2. Basal electrical activity of jejunal biopsies from control (○) and CF (●) children

Abbreviations used: PD, potential difference; R, resistance; SCC, short-circuit current. Values are mean ± S.E.; individual values are also plotted as symbols ● or ○. Significance values are control versus CF.

epithelium (see Chapter 4). As dysfunction of this transport system has been demonstrated in airway epithelium from patients with CF [3], it seems likely that such a defect might also be expressed in the enterocyte.

Chloride secretion in the intestine can be stimulated by a large number of endogenous and exogenous agents which activate the enterocyte by three main intracellular signalling systems (Fig. 4), leading to the opening of luminal chloride channels:

— (i) A change in phosphoinositide metabolism is thought to be responsible for an elevation of intracellular free calcium levels which may activate chloride channels via calmodulin and C-kinase; acetylcholine (ACh) is thought to activate this pathway.
— (ii) An increased production of cyclic AMP stimulates chloride channel opening via protein kinase A; prostaglandin E_2 (PGE_2) acts in this way.
— (iii) An increased production of cyclic GMP activates chloride channels via protein kinase G — a mechanism used by the heat-stable enterotoxin of *Escherichia coli* (*E. coli* STa).

Each of these agents (or secretagogues) increases the SCC generated by control biopsies (Fig. 5), an effect which is consistent with their ability to stimulate chloride secretion [4, 5]. This has been confirmed by the reduction of the response in chloride-free conditions. In contrast, the CF biopsies fail to respond to secretagogue challenge, indicating that the chloride secretory mechanism in the intestine, like that in the airway epithelium, is defective in CF. There are, however, some differences in that the intestine does not respond to secretagogues acting via any of the three pathways described above, while in the airway the defect seems to be specific to cyclic AMP-mediated stimulation. The response to calcium-mediated secretagogues appears unimpaired [6]. The

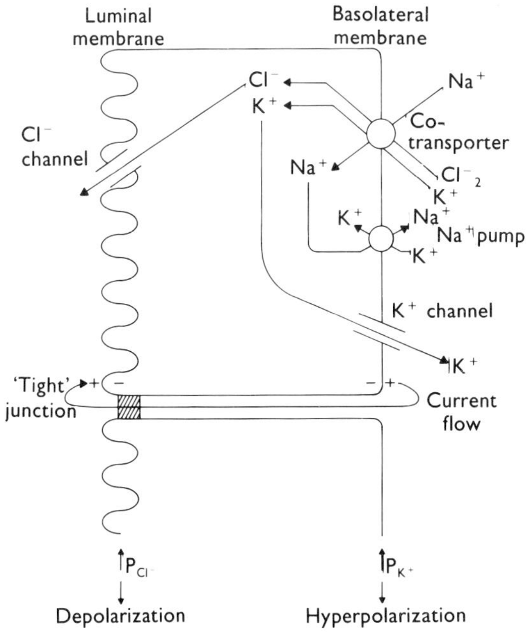

Fig. 3. Mechanism of electrogenic chloride secretion by the enterocyte

failure of the intestinal chloride secretory mechanism in CF has also been observed in larger sheets of intestinal tissue obtained during operative bowel resection, and ion flux determinations have indicated that both the stimulation of chloride secretion and the inhibition of neutral sodium chloride absorption fail in CF [7].

The failure of the intestinal secretory mechanism in CF could explain the lower basal PD and SCC in biopsies from patients with the disease. Intestinal sheets are known to exhibit a basal chloride secretion which may be related to the release of endogenous secretagogues during the mounting procedure. The absence of such endogenous chloride secretion in the CF biopsies would account for their lower basal electrical activity.

The ability of enterocytes to produce a secretory response to bacterial toxins is of considerable clinical interest. In CF biopsies, not only is the response to *E. coli* STa absent, but also that to cholera toxin [8]. In control biopsies, application of cholera toxin (50 μg/ml) to the luminal side of the tissue causes a rise in SCC of 33.8 ± 9.6 $\mu A/cm^2$ ($n=4$) after 90 min exposure, while in CF biopsies there is a fall of 10.3 ± 3.2 $\mu A/cm^2$ ($n=4$) over the same period ($P<0.01$). This would suggest that patients with CF should not suffer from secretory diarrhoea induced by bacterial toxins.

All the secretagogues discussed so far exert their effects by an interaction with receptors on the surface of the enterocyte. To test the involvement of such mechanisms in the failure of the secretory response in CF, the effects of secretagogues acting beyond these membrane receptors have been assessed. Dibutyryl cyclic AMP, which mimics the actions of endogenous cyclic AMP, produces the same pattern of results as that observed previously, where control tissues exhibit a rise in SCC while CF tissues do not (Fig. 6). This suggests that the defect in CF is located beyond the site of generation of cyclic AMP and this has been confirmed in experiments where cyclic AMP levels have been measured directly in enterocytes isolated from control and CF biopsies (Table 2). Basal cyclic AMP levels are similar in the two groups of tissues and their responses to PGE_2 and vasoactive intestinal polypeptide (VIP) are not significantly different.

The calcium ionophore, A23187, activates secretion by elevating intracellular calcium

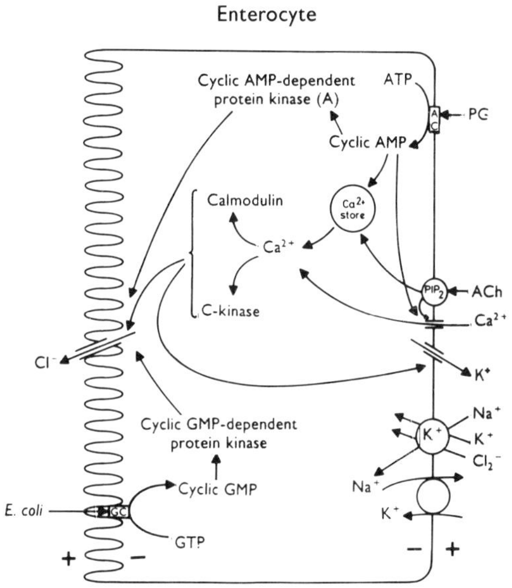

Fig. 4. Intracellular mechanisms mediating the secretory response of the enterocyte
See text for details.

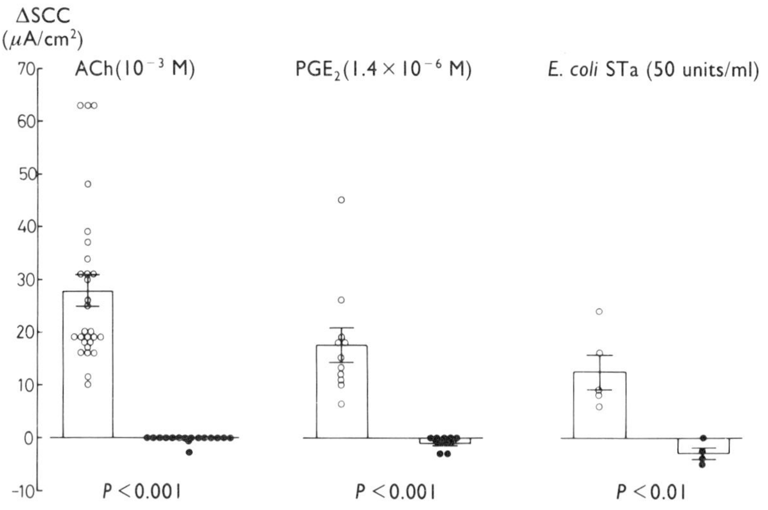

Fig. 5. Increase in SCC (ΔSCC) generated by control (○) and CF (●) jejunal biopsies in response to secretagogues acting at membrane receptors

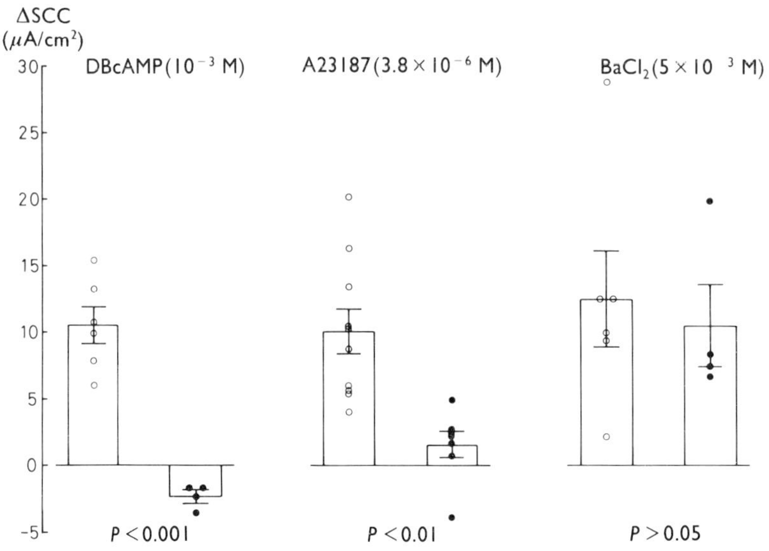

Fig. 6. Increase in SCC (ΔSCC) generated by control (○) and CF (●) jejunal biopsies in response to secretagogues acting beyond membrane receptors

Table 2 **Intracellular mediators in enterocytes isolated from jejunal biopsies from control and CF children and their response to secretagogue challenge**

Intracellular mediator	Control	CF
Cyclic AMP (fmol per 10^5 cells)		
Basal	716 ± 84 (13)	575 ± 22 (5)
VIP (10^{-7} M)	4144 ± 257 (3)**	4061 ± 98 (3)**
PGE_2 (7×10^{-6} M)	1190 ± 123 (13)*	1251 ± 213 (4)**
Intracellular free Ca^{2+} concentration (nM)		
Basal	287 ± 28 (9)	225 (1)
Ionomycin (10^{-7} M)	640 ± 17 (3)**	663 (1)

*Significance of secretagogue action: *$P < 0.01$, **$P < 0.001$. No significant difference between control and CF enterocytes under any conditions.*

directly and this is evident from the rise in SCC in control biopsies (Fig. 6). Some CF biopsies also generate an increase in SCC when the ionophore is added, although the response is smaller than in control tissues. Another way of inducing calcium-mediated intestinal secretion is to apply barium chloride which, in animal experiments, has been shown to evoke fluid and electrolyte secretion, probably by releasing calcium from intracellular stores [9]. This agent induces similar increases in SCC in control and CF tissues (Fig. 6). These findings suggest that it would be interesting to determine the changes in intracellular calcium that occur in response to secretagogue challenge in the two groups of tissues. It is possible to measure intracellular calcium levels using a fluorescent probe such as Fura 2. In chicken enterocytes this has revealed a rise in cytosolic calcium when secretagogues are added [10]. This approach has therefore been adopted in the enterocytes isolated from control and CF biopsies. With this preparation it is possible to determine basal calcium levels and to demonstrate an elevation when the calcium ionophore ionomycin is added (Table 2). Control and CF cells behave similarly in these studies. It has not proved possible, however, to demonstrate any change in calcium levels in response to secretagogues that are thought to elevate intracellular calcium via membrane receptors. Moreover, there are no reports in the literature of the successful measurement of intracellular calcium in mammalian enterocytes. Thus, the question of whether the mechanism to elevate intracellular calcium operates normally in CF remains to be answered.

- ▶ The enterocytes of the gastro-intestinal tract epithelium are involved in the transport of ions and nutrients.
- ▶ Transport across jejunal biopsies from children with CF can be measured in a modified Ussing chamber; these biopsies have a similar tissue resistance to the control, but their PD and SCC values are significantly lower.
- ▶ CF biopsies fail to respond to the secretagogues that stimulate the opening of chloride ion channels in normal intestine; this indicates that, as in the airway epithelium, the chloride ion secretory mechanism in the intestine is defective in CF.
- ▶ As basal and stimulated cyclic AMP levels are similar in both control and CF tissues, it is thought that the defect in CF is located beyond the site of cyclic AMP generation.

Secretory response of the rectal mucosa

Studies with biopsies from the rectal mucosa have revealed a similar failure of chloride secretion in this region of the intestinal tract [11]. In control tissues, ACh (10^{-3} M) and PGE_2 (1.4×10^{-6} M) increase the SCC by 83.0 ± 16.4 $\mu A/cm^2$ ($n = 12$) and 35.8 ± 14.9 $\mu A/cm^2$

($n = 11$), respectively, but such responses are absent in tissues from children with CF, although both groups exhibit a similar fall in SCC with the inhibitor of electrogenic sodium absorption, 10^{-4} M amiloride [control, $-37.7 \pm 7.7(12)$ $\mu A/cm^2$; CF, $-44.0 \pm 9.3(5)$ $\mu A/cm^2$].

Secretory response *in vivo*

In vitro studies have established that the chloride secretory mechanism of both the small and large intestine fails to operate in CF. To determine whether this defect is observed *in vivo*, the secretory response can be measured in adult volunteers, using a rise in the transintestinal PD as an index of chloride secretion [12]. A multi-lumen tube is introduced so that its tip is located in the proximal jejunum. One lumen of the tube is connected to a pressure transducer to record intraluminal pressure and another to a salt bridge electrode to record the PD. A second salt bridge electrode is applied subcutaneously and both electrodes are connected via calomel half cells to a battery-powered electrometer with a visual record being displayed on a multichannel chart recorder. Secretion can be stimulated by intraluminal application of the cholinergic agonist pilocarpine and by PGE_2. In control subjects these secretagogues induce a rise in PD, but

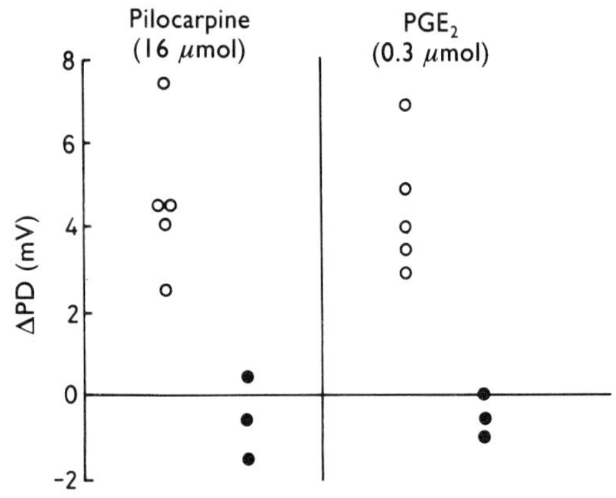

Fig. 7. Increase in transintestinal PD (ΔPD) induced by pilocarpine and PGE_2 in the jejunum of normal (○) and CF (●) adult volunteers

this response is absent in the CF patients (Fig. 7). A similar study in the rectum has also demonstrated that the rise in PD induced by theophylline, which acts via cyclic AMP, fails to occur in subjects with CF [13]. Thus, the defect observed *in vitro* is a reflection of the situation *in vivo*. These experiments also provide an opportunity to examine the relationship between the transintestinal PD and motility. It has been reported that an increase in motor activity is associated with a rise in the transintestinal PD and this was attributed to a stimulation of chloride secretion [14]. Because of the transient nature of the response it was not possible to demonstrate this directly. The fact that chloride secretion does not occur in CF patients allows this hypothesis to be tested. Recordings of PD and intraluminal pressure from the jejunum of a control and a CF subject are shown in Fig. 8. An increase in motor activity in the control subject is accompanied by a rise in the PD of about 10 mV in amplitude. The increased motor activity in the CF subject, however, is not associated with any alteration in the PD. This strongly supports the contention that the rise in PD that accompanies increased motility in normal subjects does indeed represent chloride secretion.

The *in vivo* studies confirm the *in vitro* data which indicate that the intestinal secretory response is absent in CF. It is therefore possible to make use of this distinction as an aid to diagnosis in cases where the sweat test is impractical or unacceptable, or produces ambiguous results [12, 15].

Secretory response in heterozygotes

The secretory response of heterozygotes has also been examined using the *in vivo* technique. The high incidence of the CF gene in the population has long been a subject for speculation as it was assumed that heterozygotes must possess some survival advantage, although the nature of this was obscure. Examination of the intestinal secretory response to pilocarpine, however, reveals a significant difference between heterozygotes and normals, with heterozygotes exhibiting a reduced response (Fig. 9) indicating a degree of expression of the CF gene. If this difference is translated into a blunted response to the diarrhoeagenic action

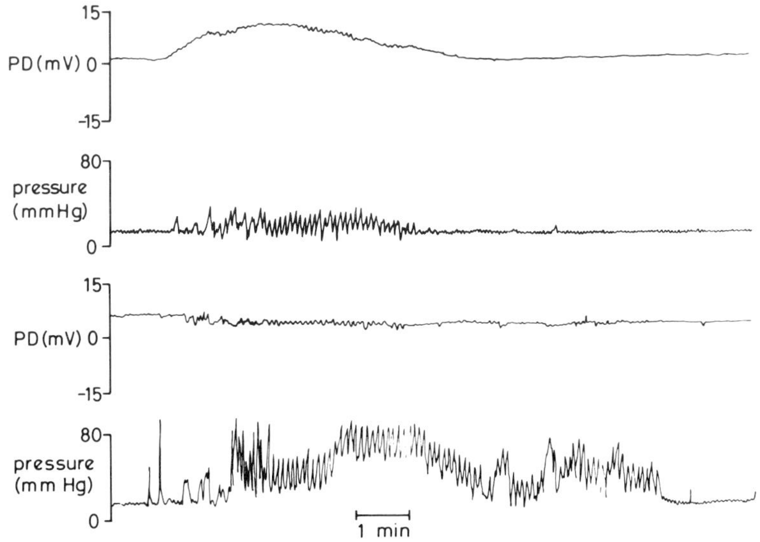

Fig. 8. Transintestinal PD and intraluminal pressure recordings from the jejunum of a normal subject (upper trace) and of a CF patient (lower trace)

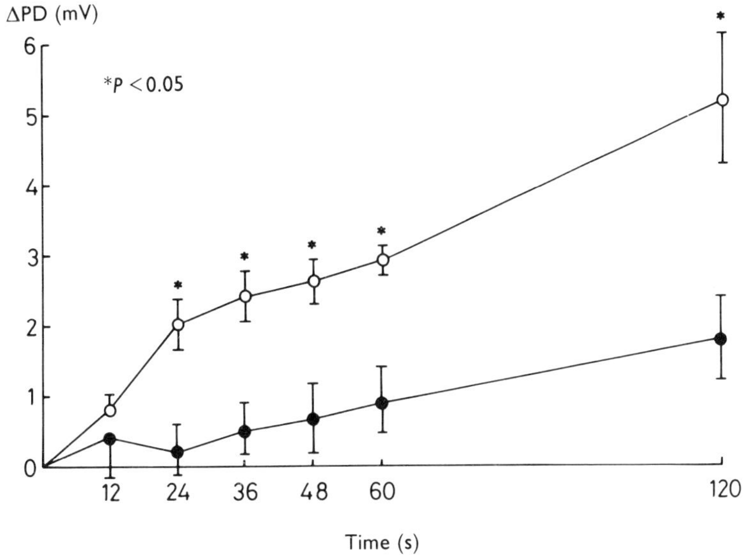

Fig. 9. Change in transintestinal PD (ΔPD) induced by pilocarpine (16 μmol) in five normal subjects (○) and 10 heterozygotes carrying the CF gene (●)
** Indicates a significant difference between the two groups.*

of bacterial toxins, this could well represent a survival advantage, as, historically, diarrhoeal disease is a major cause of death. Such an effect could therefore explain the prevalence of the CF gene.

Nutrient absorption

As well as its secretory function, the intestine is also concerned with the absorption of nutrients. It was reported some years ago that the absorption of glucose was enhanced in CF [16]. This was based on *in vivo* studies, and so it was not possible to distinguish between effects on the active or passive components of glucose uptake. Using the Ussing chamber technique it is possible to focus on the active component, since the rise in SCC that occurs when glucose is added to the luminal fluid is a reflection of its active absorption. Glucose enters the enterocyte against its concentration gradient using energy from the sodium gradient, harnessed by a coupled carrier located in the luminal membrane (Fig. 10). The sodium ions that enter with the glucose are removed from the cell by the basolateral sodium pump and it is this increased movement of sodium from mucosa to serosa that is responsible for the rise in SCC associated with the absorption of glucose and other actively transported nutrients. The ability of biopsies from both control and CF children to actively absorb glucose is demonstrated by the rise in PD and SCC that occurs when glucose (10 mM) is added to the luminal solution. This is a useful test of viability in the CF tissues which fail to give a response to secretory stimulants. When

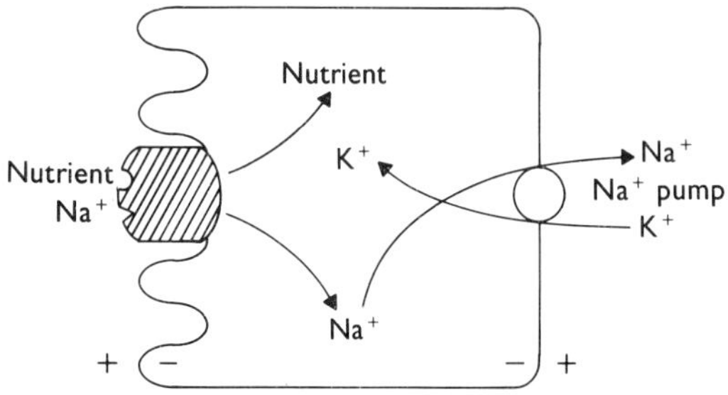

Fig. 10. Mechanism of active nutrient absorption by the enterocyte

the data is analysed it is evident that the magnitude of the glucose-dependent rise in SCC is greater in the CF biopsies [41.2 ± 5.8 $\mu A/cm^2$ ($n = 17$)] than it is in the controls [22.4 ± 3.0 $\mu A/cm^2$ ($n = 28$), $P < 0.01$] and this effect is observed over a range of concentrations (Fig. 11).

The addition of glucose to the luminal solution not only initiates absorption of the sugar, but also exerts an osmotic gradient which can itself influence transintestinal electrical activity. To compensate for this effect, control experiments must be carried out using equimolar mannitol. This induces a fall in SCC which is greater in the CF tissues (Fig. 11). The change in electrical activity induced by the osmotic gradient has several components. The resulting movement of water across the tissue generates a profile asymmetry potential due to the distortion of ion profiles within the membrane; it displaces mobile ions through charged junctions, and it generates a boundary diffusion potential due to the dilution of fluid immediately adjacent to the membrane. This latter action could be influenced by the absence of chloride permeability in the luminal membrane of CF enterocytes. Dilution of the fluid adjacent to the luminal membrane will lead to its hyperpolarization with a consequent decrease in the transepithelial PD and SCC. In normal cells the magnitude of this effect would be reduced by a significant chloride permeability which would allow a depolarizing efflux of chloride ions across the luminal membrane. The absence of such chloride movement in CF cells would enhance any osmotically induced hyperpolarization, thus accounting for the greater reduction in transepithelial electrical activity induced by luminal mannitol in CF biopsies. When the osmotic effect is taken into account, the difference between control and CF tissues with respect to glucose absorption is even more pronounced. A kinetic analysis of the data indicates that there is an increase in the maximum capacity of the transport system, an effect that is also observed with the actively transported amino acid, alanine [17].

Conclusions

The intestine of patients with CF not only fails to secrete chloride, but, in the case of the small bowel, also possesses an enhanced capacity for

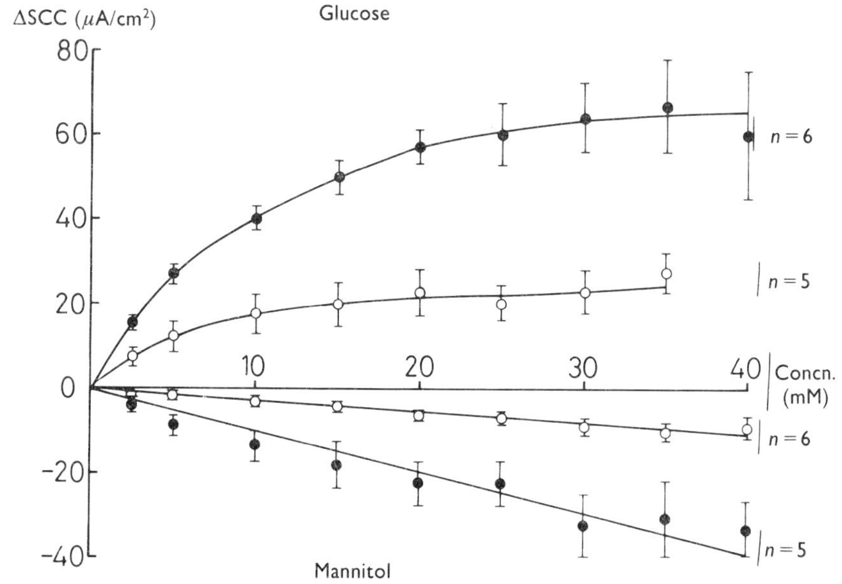

Fig. 11. Change in SCC (ΔSCC) induced by increasing concentrations of glucose and mannitol in jejunal biopsies from control (○) and CF (●) children

Note that the increase in SCC induced by glucose is enhanced in CF, as is the decrease produced by mannitol.

the active absorption of nutrients. As water follows net solute movement this will lead to a relative dehydration of the luminal contents with a consequent tendency to obstruction. Since CF is a single gene defect, all the symptoms of the disease should be attributed to a common cause. In the case of the changes in intestinal transport, both the absence of secretion and the enhanced absorption can be explained in terms of a failure in the mechanism for opening the chloride channels in the luminal membrane of the enterocyte (Fig. 12). These chloride channels are an integral part of the secretory mechanism and so their failure to open in response to stimulation accounts for the absence of a secretory response in CF. In normal cells, chloride permeability will depolarize the luminal membrane, thus reducing the driving force for sodium-linked nutrient entry. In CF cells this depolarizing action of chloride ions will be absent and hence there will be an enhanced sodium gradient for nutrient uptake. Alternatively the defect in CF could reside in a regulatory factor that influences more than one ion transport mechanism, and which, in the enterocyte, may act independently on chloride secretion and sodium-linked nutrient absorption.

The fact that the intestine expresses the defect in chloride channel operation that is characteristic of CF means that this tissue can be used both to investigate the basic defect and to test the effects of potential therapeutic agents. In addition, the clear distinction between the secretory response of control and CF biopsies could be used to confirm the diagnosis of the disease in cases where sweat test results are ambiguous.

The reason for this failure in the operation of chloride channels in CF is not yet fully understood. Recently, the CF gene has been identified and the amino acid composition of the gene product, the so-called CF transmembrane conductance regulator (CFTR), is now known [18]. This has several sequences that are similar to those found in transmembrane proteins, leading to the suggestion that the CFTR may represent the chloride channel regulator. In 70% of CF patients the defective gene results in the deletion of a single amino acid, phenylalanine in position 508, from the gene product. The site of this deletion is one of the nucleotide-binding folds which supports the idea that it is the regulatory mechanism that controls the chloride channel that is defective in CF. The discovery of the gene should produce exciting developments in our understanding of the defect in CF with the possibility that this could lead to an effective therapy for the treatment of the disease.

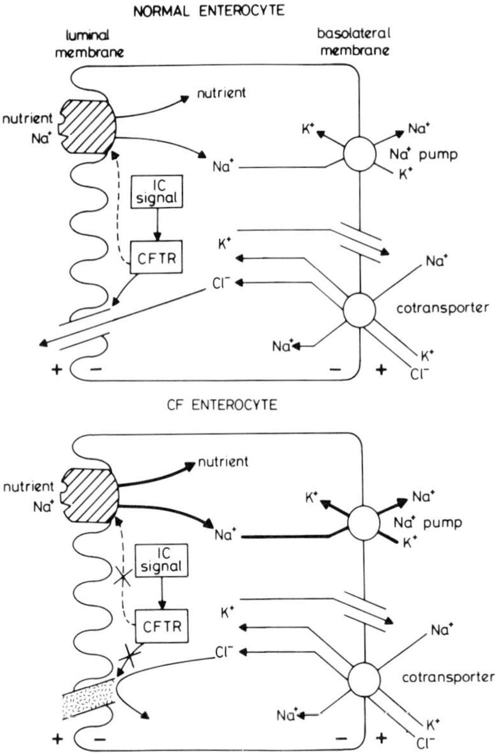

Fig. 12. Model to explain the changes in intestinal transport that occur in CF

In the normal enterocyte, secretagogue challenge generates an intracellular (IC) signal which acts via the cystic fibrosis transmembrane conductance regulator (CFTR) to open chloride channels in the luminal membrane. The resulting chloride efflux may reduce the electrochemical gradient for sodium-linked nutrient entry. In the CF enterocyte, a defect in the CFTR leads to the failure of chloride channels to open when stimulated and is responsible for the loss of the secretory response. It may also cause a reduction in the depolarization of the luminal membrane, leading to enhanced nutrient absorption. Alternatively CFTR could regulate sodium-linked nutrient uptake independently (----). Potassium channel function in CF enterocytes has not yet been investigated and it is assumed that, as in the airway, it is normal.

At present, therapy is directed towards ameliorating the symptoms of CF rather than correcting the basic defect. Progressive lung disease, from recurrent endobronchial infection, can be reduced by regular physiotherapy and antibiotics. The majority of CF patients also require pancreatic enzyme supplements to improve the absorption of nutrients. Enzymes are inactivated by gastric acid but can be given enclosed in acid-resistant microspheres, allowing the release of active enzymes in the duodenum. Histamine H_2 receptor antagonists may also be used to reduce gastric acid secretion and thus enhance the function of both enzymes and bile salts.

Obstruction of the bowel by dehydrated sticky contents — meconium ileus — occurs in the newborn. Osmotically active agents, such as X-ray contrast media, can be instilled into the rectum to rehydrate the intestinal contents, but failure to then pass meconium necessitates urgent surgical relief of the blockage with resection of the obstructed segment of bowel and a temporary ileostomy. A similar problem — distal ileal obstruction syndrome (DIOS) — can be seen in older children and CF adults. This usually responds to osmotically active agents given orally and recurrence can often be prevented by improving control of fat absorption with additional pancreatic enzymes.

It is possible that, in the future, gene therapy may be used to correct the basic defect of CF; i.e. the insertion of genes coding for the production of normal CFTR into affected cells might restore effective regulation of ion transport.

► Using a rise in the transintestinal PD as an index, *in vivo* studies confirm the *in vitro* data that the intestinal secretory response is absent in CF; thus, the distinction can be used as an aid to diagnosis in cases where the sweat test is impractical.

► In addition to the failure of chloride secretion in CF, active nutrient absorption is enhanced, exacerbating the dehydration of the luminal contents of the intestine.

► In 70% of CF patients, the defective gene results in the deletion of a single amino acid within one of the nucleotide-binding folds of CFTR; this suggests that it is the regulatory mechanism controlling the chloride channel that is defective in CF.
► Although, at present, treatment of CF is directed towards ameliorating the symptoms, it may become possible, in the future, to correct the basic gene defect using gene therapy.

We gratefully acknowledge the contributions made by other members of the CF Group in Sheffield (Prof. B. L. Brown, Prof. N. W. Read, Dr P. S. Baxter, Dr P. M. Dobson, Dr B. W. Hitchin, Dr A. J. Wilson and Mr J. Goldhill). We also wish to thank the Cystic Fibrosis Research Trust and Janssen Pharmaceutica for financial support.

References

1. Bukhave, K. and Rask-Madsen, J. (1980) Saturation kinetics applied to *in vitro* effects of low prostaglandin E_2 and $F_{2\alpha}$ concentrations on ion transport across human jejunal mucosa. Gastroenterology **78**, 32–42
2. Hardcastle, J. and Hardcastle, P. T. (1987) Membrane permeability changes in intestinal secretion. Med. Sci. Res. **15**, 471–473
3. Welsh, M. J. and Fick, R. B. (1987) Cystic fibrosis. J. Clin. Invest. **80**, 1523–1526
4. Taylor, C. J., Baxter, P. S., Hardcastle, J. and Hardcastle, P. T. (1987) Absence of secretory response in jejunal biopsy samples from children with cystic fibrosis. Lancet **II**, 107–108
5. Taylor, C. J., Baxter, P. S., Hardcastle, J. and Hardcastle, P. T. (1988) Failure to induce secretion in jejunal biopsies from children with cystic fibrosis. Gut **29**, 957–962
6. Boucher, R. C., Cheng, E. H. C., Paradiso, A. M., Stutts, M. J., Knowles, M. R. and Earp, H. S. (1989) Chloride secretory response of cystic fibrosis human airway epithelia. J. Clin. Invest. **84**, 1424–1431
7. Berschneider, H. M., Knowles, M. R., Azizkhan, R. G., Boucher, R. C., Tobey, N. A., Orlando, R. C. and Powell, D. W. (1988) Altered intestinal chloride transport in cystic fibrosis. FASEB J. **2**, 2625–2629
8. Baxter, P. S., Goldhill, J., Hardcastle, J., Hardcastle, P. T. and Taylor, C. J. (1988) Accounting for cystic fibrosis. Nature (London) **335**, 211
9. Hardcastle, J., Hardcastle, P. T. and Noble, J. M. (1983) The effect of barium chloride on intestinal secretion in the rat. J Physiol. **344**, 69–80
10. Chang, E. B., Brown, D. R., Wang, N. S. and Field, M. (1986) Secretagogue-induced changes in membrane calcium permeability in chicken and chinchilla ileal mucosa. J. Clin. Invest. **78**, 281–287
11. Hardcastle, J., Hardcastle, P. T., Taylor, C. J. and Goldhill, J. (1991) Failure of cholinergic stimulation to induce a secretory response from the rectal mucosa in cystic fibrosis. Gut **32**, 1035–1039
12. Baxter, P. S., Wilson, A. J., Read, N. W., Hardcastle, J., Hardcastle, P. T. and Taylor, C. J. (1989) Abnormal jejunal potential difference in cystic fibrosis. Lancet **I**, 464–466
13. Goldstein, J. L., Nash, N. T., Al-Bazzaz, F., Layden, T. J. and Rao, M. C. (1988) Rectum has abnormal ion transport but normal cAMP-binding proteins in cystic fibrosis. Am. J. Physiol. **254**, C719–C724
14. Read, N. W., Smallwood, R. H., Levin, R. J., Holdsworth, C. D. and Brown, B. H. (1977) Relationship between change in intraluminal pressure and transmural potential difference in the human and canine jejunum *in vivo*. Gut **18**, 141–151
15. Taylor, C. J., Baxter, P. S., Hardcastle, J., Hardcastle, P. T. and Goldhill, J. (1990) New diagnostic method for cystic fibrosis. Acta Universitatis Carolinae Medica **36**, 142–143
16. Frase, L. L., Strickland, A. D., Kachel, G. W. and Krejs, G. J. (1985) Enhanced glucose absorption in the jejunum of patients with cystic fibrosis. Gastroenterology **88**, 478–484
17. Baxter, P. S., Goldhill, J., Hardcastle, J., Hardcastle, P. T. and Taylor, C. J. (1990) Enhanced intestinal glucose and alanine transport in cystic fibrosis. Gut **31**, 817–820
18. Riordan, J. R., Rommens, J. M., Kerem, B.-S., Alon, N., Rozmahel, R., Grzelczak, Z., Zielenski, J., Lok, S., Plavsic, N., Chou, J.-L., Drumm, M. L., Iannuzzi, M. C., Collins, F. S. and Tsui, L.-C. (1989) Identification of the cystic fibrosis gene: cloning and characterization of complementary DNA. Science **245**, 1067–1072

6

Hypersecretion in the airways

Niels Mygind
Otopathological Laboratory, Department of Otolaryngology and Allergy Clinic, Department of Medicine TTA, Righospitalet, DK-2100 Copenhagen, Denmark

Introduction

The clinical consequences of hypersecretion in the upper and lower airways are nasal discharge, sputum production and, in some cases, airways obstruction. Diseases associated with these symptoms include allergic and non-allergic rhinitis, common cold and other acute airway infections, asthma, chronic bronchitis, cystic fibrosis and primary ciliary dyskinesia. In addition, plugging of the lower airways by stagnant secretions is an important cause of infection, atelectasis and respiratory failure in severely ill and intubated patients.

This chapter will address the pathogenic mechanisms of airway hypersecretion. However, three major problems are associated with this topic. First, we cannot measure the secretory rate in living humans, which makes a definition of hypersecretion difficult. Second, the surface liquid in the airways is a mixture of a secretory product from glands and goblet cells and of liquid from other sources. Third, accumulation of surface liquids depends not only upon production rate but also upon removal (mucociliary function).

Airway mucus

Mucous membranes are so named because of their capacity to secrete mucus, and the liquid collected from the surface of the conducting airways is called 'mucus' or 'airway secretion', although non-secretory products, derived from plasma, surface epithelial cells, and cell debris, contribute to its volume and properties.

Airway mucus in healthy subjects is composed of water (95%), mucus glycoproteins or mucins (2%), other proteins including albumin, immunoglobulins, lysozyme and lactoferrin (1%), inorganic salts (1%) and lipids (<1%) [1].

The submucosal glands, and to a lesser degree the goblet cells, are the main source of mucus glycoproteins that provide mucus with its characteristic viscoelastic properties. The mucus glycoproteins consist of a protein core (20%) with oligosaccharide side chains (80%) [2], crosslinked by disulphide and hydrogen bonds (Fig. 1).

The concentration of mucus glycoproteins cannot be measured directly in a sample of air-

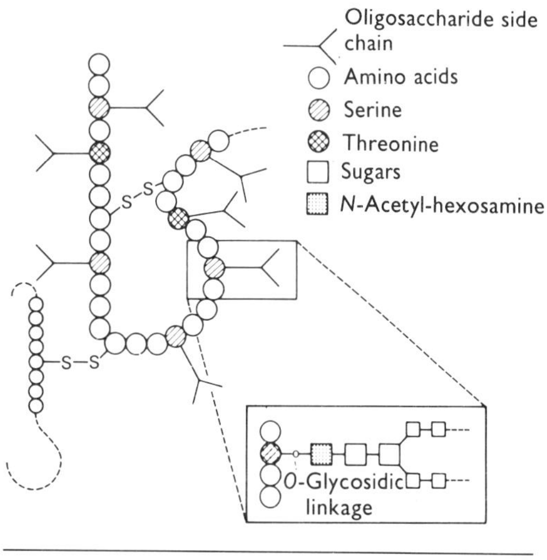

Fig. 1. Schematic structure of human airway mucus glycoproteins, which consist of a protein core, rich in serine and threonine
Attached to the protein core are oligosaccharide side chains linked via an O-glycosidic bond between either serine or threonine on the protein core and N-acetylgalactosamine on the oligosaccharide side chain. There are intrachain and interchain disulphide linkages as well. Reproduced from [2] with permission.

way fluid, but fucose can be used as a marker of mucus glycoproteins, and mannose of plasma glycoproteins [3].

The mucus from glands contains in addition proteins secreted by the serous acini. These proteins (e.g. secretory-immunoglobulin A, lysozyme, lactoferrin and antileukoprotease) play a defensive role against infectious agents [4, 5].

Mucus can cross-link and produce a viscoelastic gel that can form a mechanical coupling with cilia and be transported by them. Nasal secretions have a considerably lower viscosity than tracheobronchial secretions, but a comparable elasticity [6], and elasticity is more important than viscosity for mucus transport. In purulent secretions, a high content of plasma proteins, and of DNA from neutrophils, will add to the viscosity of the secretion.

As mentioned earlier, the secretory rate in the airways cannot be measured in humans *in vivo*. The total net volume passing through the trachea has been estimated to be 10 ml/day. This rough estimate is based on sampling from tracheotomized patients [7]. Using fine micropipettes, the resting secretion from a single airway gland in cat trachea has been measured to be 9 nl/min [8]. A maximally stimulated human nose can produce about 5 ml/h.

Clinical data indicate that there is a diurnal variation in the nose with reduced secretion rate at night [9]. In the tracheobronchial tree the clearance of secretions is markedly reduced during sleep [10]; this may contribute to the early morning cough, sputum and wheeziness in many patients.

Mucociliary system

The mucous membrane from the nose to the alveoli is covered by cilia (Fig. 2). These are 0.3 μm in diameter and 5 μm long. Each cell is covered by approximately 100 cilia, which beat in a synchronous way with a frequency of 1000 strokes per minute (Fig. 3). The direction of beating is backwards in the nose and upwards in the tracheobronchial tree. In this way, the cilia convey the mucus with its trapped inhaled particles, micro-organisms and cellular debris to the throat where it is swallowed.

The mucus layer is probably a double layer, consisting of an aqueous periciliary sol phase in which the cilia beat, and a superficial blanket of gel which is moved forwards by the tips of the cilia [11]. Both layers are about 5 μm thick.

It is remarkable that the thin covering layer can be kept at a constant thickness during its movement from the peripheral airways to the trachea, as the total cross-sectional circum-

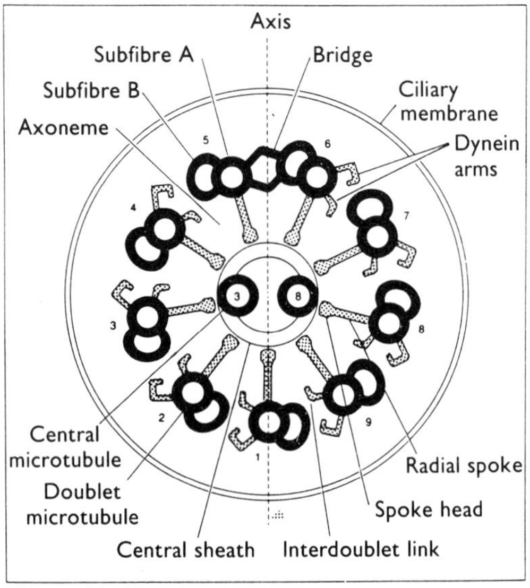

Fig 2. Diagram of a cilium cross-section, viewed from the base towards the tip
A ring of nine doublet microtubules surrounds two single central microtubules. Each doublet microtubule has two subfibres, A and B: dynein arms project from subfibre A towards the next microtubule's subfibre B. Reprinted with permission from [51].

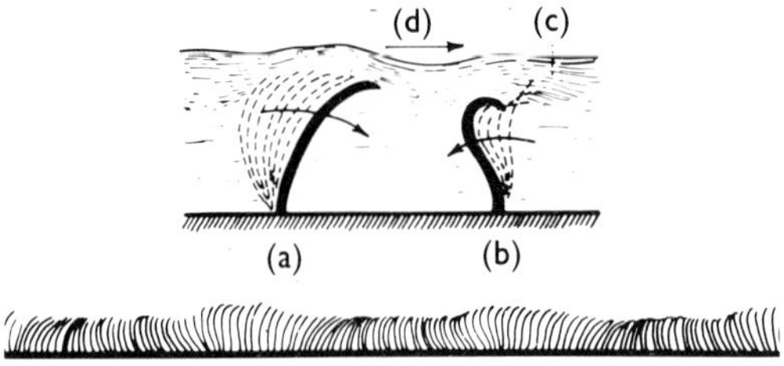

Fig. 3. Diagram showing the character of ciliary beating
Each cilium beats with an effective stroke **(a)** *and a recovery stroke* **(b)**. *The mucus blanket* **(c)** *is always moved in the same direction as the effective stroke* **(d)**. *Metachronal waves are shown in the lower part of the Figure. Reprinted with permission from [52].*

ference changes from many metres to a few centimetres. This must require active absorption of electrolytes and water over the surface epithelium. Thus, the volume of the surface liquid in the airways reflects a balance between secretion and absorption, but the exact mechanism behind this fine regulation remains largely unknown [12, 13].

The thickness and composition of the double layer is important for mucociliary transport. If the sol layer is too thin, ciliary beating will be inhibited by the viscous surface layer. If it is too thick, the gel layer loses its contact with the cilia and mucociliary clearance is impaired (Fig. 4).

Mucociliary transport rate will also depend upon the number of ciliated cells (reduced in common cold and chronic bronchitis), and the co-ordination of ciliary beating (abnormal in primary ciliary dyskinesia).

Submucosal glands

Normal airway glands are all formed in foetal life [14], which indicates that the newborn has a relatively high secretory capacity, when the number of glands is related to the area of the ciliated surface. However, formation of acini, and thereby growth of the glandular mass, occurs mainly after birth. In airways disease, such as chronic bronchitis, the number of glands remains constant [14], but the total glandular mass can be enlarged [15]. There can be a new formation of glands during chronic infection in some tissues (paranasal sinuses, middle ear) [14]. However, as these glands are not innervated, they are structurally and functionally abnormal, and they will undergo cystic degeneration [16].

There are submucosal (seromucous) glands in the nose, pharynx, larynx, trachea and bronchi, i.e. in the cartilagenous parts of the airways.

A submucosal gland consists of a central excretory duct which divides dichotonously into collecting tubules, which end in seromucous acini. The luminal part of the excretory duct is covered by cilia (Fig. 4), which assist in the expulsion of mucus from the opening of the duct. The presence of a large number of mitochondria in the duct cells suggests that active

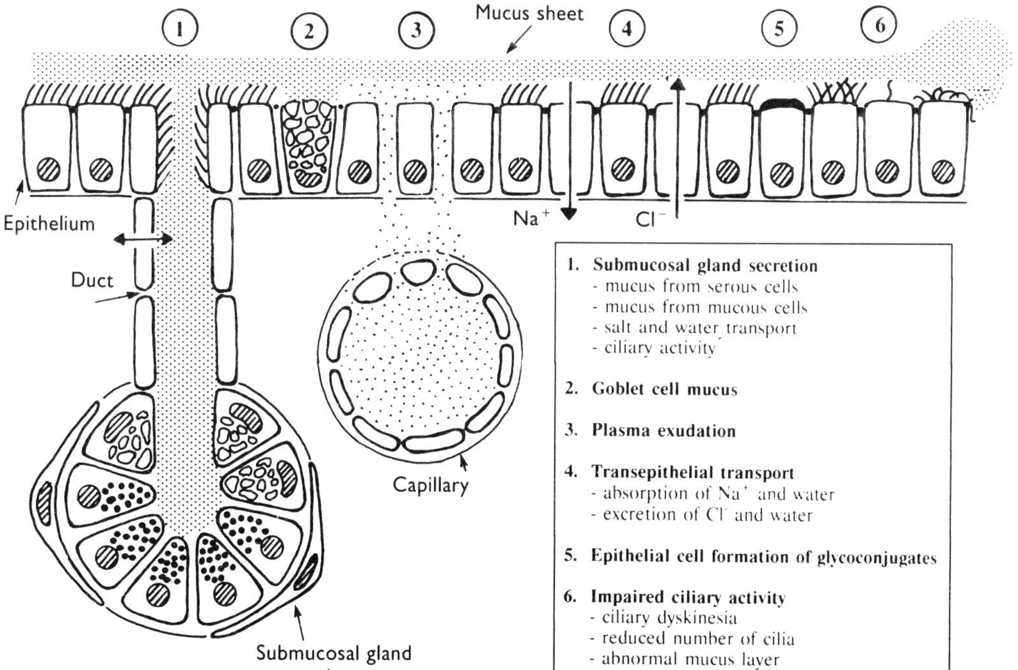

1. **Submucosal gland secretion**
   - mucus from serous cells
   - mucus from mucous cells
   - salt and water transport
   - ciliary activity
2. **Goblet cell mucus**
3. **Plasma exudation**
4. **Transepithelial transport**
   - absorption of Na^+ and water
   - excretion of Cl^- and water
5. **Epithelial cell formation of glycoconjugates**
6. **Impaired ciliary activity**
   - ciliary dyskinesia
   - reduced number of cilia
   - abnormal mucus layer

Fig. 4. Sources of airway surface liquids

metabolism, and probably transepithelial electrolyte secretion with passive diffusion of water, control the hydration of the final secretory product [17].

In the secretory acini, the mucous cells are located in the proximal and serous cells in the distal portion (Fig. 4). This explains the histologically described 'serous halfmoons' seen in a cross-section of an acinus. The mucous and serous cells have the same ultrastructural characteristics as similar cell types in other glands in the body.

An acinus is surrounded by myoepithelial cells (Fig. 4), which probably play a role in secretory cell discharge. The osmotic effect of secreted glycoproteins from mucous and serous cells and of proteins from serous cells may also be important for the passive diffusion of water and, consequently, for the volume of secretion [4, 5]. However, our knowledge of the secretory mechanisms and their regulation under various conditions is incomplete.

The serous cells dominate in the nose (90% of acini; N. Mygind, unpublished work) and, to a lesser extent, also in the bronchial tree (60% of gland volume) [18].

In the nose, there are 90 000 glands (eight per mm^2), in the pharynx 1100 and in the trachea 4000 (one per mm^2); a tracheal gland has three times the volume of a nasal gland [19]. The glandular density and size decrease in the bronchi, and the glands disappear together with the cartilage. Thus, the nose probably has a higher mucus-producing capacity per mm^2 than the tracheobronchial tree.

In the normal tracheobronchial tree the total volume of the submucosal glands has been estimated to be 4 ml, or about 40 times greater than that of the surface mucous cells (goblet cells) [20]. There is the same relative dominance of glandular cells in the nose, while goblet cells dominate in the paranasal sinuses (and middle ear), which normally have very few glands [14].

► Mucus is secreted from the mucous membrane; it is composed primarily of water with a small percentage of glycoproteins (mucin).
► The submucosal glands and, to a lesser extent, the goblet cells (surface mucous cells) are the main source of mucus glycoproteins.

► Submucosal glands reside in all cartilagenous parts of the airways; in airways disease, these may increase in mass.
► The cilia of the mucous membrane convey the mucus with its trapped inhaled particles, micro-organisms and cellular debris to the throat where it is swallowed.

Control of glandular mucus production

Submucosal glands produce the major part of mucus in the airways. The glands are under the control of the parasympathetic nervous system, but the significance of this system in airway disease in man seems less obvious than in animal studies. Recently, experimental studies have revealed a number of other means of stimulating the glands (outlined below), but their importance in human disease remains to be established.

Cholinergic nervous system

There is a dense cholinergic innervation of airway glands, and cholinergic nerve endings are 10 times more frequent than adrenergic nerve endings [21]. Stimulation of the parasympathetic fibres results in the secretion of fluid in most animal species [8], and the muscarinic receptor agonist acetylcholine releases mucus glycoproteins and contracts myoepithelial cells [17]. In man, inhalation of acetylcholine (or methacholine) induces sputum production [20], and nasal administration of the same results in measurable amounts of nasal secretion [22].

Parasympathetic fibres are part of a reflex arc with afferent fibres in the trigeminal nerves (nose) and the vagus nerves (tracheobronchial tree). Mechanical or chemical stimulations (e.g. histamine, 5-hydroxytryptamine, kinins, SO_2, cold air, hypertonic saline) result in glandular hypersecretion. Reflex-induced secretion from the nose is watery, but it has a content of glycoproteins, qualititatively similar to that of the more viscous tracheobronchial secretion (N. Mygind, unpublished work). The contribution of reflex-mediated secretion can be evaluated by the effect of cholinergic receptor antagonists (e.g. atropine sulphate, ipratropium bromide), which inhibit the secretion by blockage of the glandular cholinoceptors. Baseline secretion from the glands is not completely under cholinergic control because atropine can reduce but not abolish resting secretion [4, 5].

Adrenergic nervous system

While there is clear evidence of parasympathetic control of airway glands, the role of adrenergic nerves and their relationship with the mucus-secreting glands is less clear. Animal models and *in vitro* experiments with human tissue have shown that adrenoceptor agonists can stimulate airway glands. The α-receptor agonists preferentially deplete serous cells and produce copious secretions with a low viscosity, while the β-adrenoceptor agonists deplete mucous cells and produce scanty secretions with a high viscosity [23, 24].

However, daily use of α-adrenoceptor agonists as vasoconstrictors in the nose, and of β-adrenoceptor agonists as bronchodilators in the bronchi, does not appear to have a significant effect on volume or viscoelastic properties of airway secretions. Thus, extrapolation of the experimental findings to human pathophysiology needs to be carried out with caution.

Neuropeptides

In addition to the classic neurotransmitters, acetylcholine and noradrenaline, both parasympathetic and sympathetic nerves produce neuropeptides. The exact role of this class of non-adrenergic non-cholinergic (NANC) neurons in human disease is poorly understood, because adequate antagonists to the neuropeptides are not available for study.

The peptide best studied is substance P (SP). It is present in a subtype of sensory nerves, called C-fibres, and it can be released by mechanical and chemical stimulation (e.g. tobacco smoke, capsaicin, kinins, histamine). SP has many effects in the airways, including stimulation of mucus secretion and of epithelial ion transport, and it increases vascular permeability [25–28]. The term 'neurogenic inflammation' is used for the phenomenon of stimulated sensory nerves causing a tissue response by release of neuropeptides.

SP belongs to a group of neuropeptides designated tachykinins. The tachykinin response in the airways is regulated by endogenous proteases [25]. Thus, the entire system becomes more and more complicated. In addition, the effect of SP on mucus cells is species-dependent.

Vasoactive intestinal polypeptide is co-localized with acetylcholine in the cholinergic nerve endings to the glands and may possibly modulate the response to released acetylcholine. For more details about the rapidly increasing number of neuropeptides, the reader is referred to Chapter 2.

Axon reflexes

Stimulation of C-fibre sensory nerves initiates an axon reflex (intra-airway reflex running in one neuron; see Chapter 2). Experimental data suggest that C-fibres and axon reflexes can activate mucus-producing cells and induce extravasation of plasma proteins, at least in some animal species [17]. It has been suggested that C-fibres are easily stimulated in diseases characterized by damage of the airway epithelium, and that they play a role in the pathogenesis of bronchial asthma, where shedding of the surface epithelium results in exposure to free C-fibre endings that can then be more easily activated by inhalants and inflammatory mediators [29].

The distinction between two subsets of sensory nerves in the conducting airways [rapidly adapting irritant receptors involved in central nervous system (CNS) reflexes and capasicin-sensitive C-fibres involved in axon reflexes] is not definite and exclusive, as capsaicin stimulation of human nasal mucosa results in nasal discharge, and a CNS reflex response blocked by atropine [30].

Inflammatory secretagogues

A variety of cells — mast cells, eosinophils, neutrophils, lymphocytes, monocytes and macrophages — are recruited to the airways during inflammatory reactions. Upon activation, these cells release biochemical mediators which contribute to the inflammatory reaction. The role of a number of these cell-derived mediators in the stimulation of respiratory mucus production has been studied recently.

At micromolar (10^{-6} M) concentrations, histamine, prostaglandins and, in particular, leukotrienes and platelet-activating factor, release glycoproteins from human bronchial explants [17]. Some of these substances (prostaglandins and other derivatives of arachidonic acid) can also be released from activated epithelial cells [31]. Inflammatory secretagogues probably play a role in mucus production in airway inflammation, but the mechanisms by which secretagogues induce mucus secretion, and the magnitude of the effects, are unknown.

Vascular leakage occurs as a result of inflammatory processes and may contribute to the volume of airway fluid. The exudation may also expose airway secretory cells to plasma secretagogues [17].

In addition, bacterial products (e.g. elastase from *Pseudomonas aeruginosa*) can act as secretagogues.

It should be stressed that many of these data are derived from *in vitro* studies of human and experimental animal tissues. Ultimately, the relative importance of these mediators will be determined in human trials with specific antagonists.

Goblet cells

Surface mucous cells or goblet cells are present in the entire airway epithelium, including paranasal sinuses and middle ear. The number falls from 10000 per mm^2 in the nose to 7000 per mm^2 in the small airways [14], where the goblet cells in the periphery are replaced by Clara cells, which probably also have a secretory function.

Goblet cells resemble the mucous cells in the glands, but they lack innervation. Apparently, they release their content of mucus upon direct stimulation from irritant gases (e.g. SO_2), bacterial products and inflammatory mediators. It is not known how often or how many times the goblet cells can discharge mucus, how mucus production is regulated, or for how long the cells live.

The goblet cell number can be increased in persons working in a dusty atmosphere, in smokers and in patients with chronic bronchitis [14, 32]. Experimental goblet cell hyperplasia can be induced by treatment of the tissue with elastase from neutrophils [17].

Plasma exudation

Intranasal spraying of histamine and of allergen induces a prompt and transient plasma exudation with a large unfiltered bulk flow of plasma across the endothelial and epithelial barriers into the airway lumen [33, 34] (Fig. 4). Histamine causes a contraction of endothelial cells so that plasma leakage takes place as a result of an opening of the intercellular junctions. The epithelial passage of extravasated plasma is probably achieved by hydrostatic pressure on the basal side of the epithelial lining [35]. Plasma exudation, measured by albumin concentration in lavage fluid, occurs in allergic rhinitis and in asthma, and it is reduced by glucocorticoid treatment. Plasma exudation has been suggested as a pathogenic factor in the allergic inflammatory airways diseases, i.e. allergic rhinits and asthma [36, 37].

Epithelial ion and water transport

Transepithelial passage of electrolytes and water occurs in the airway epithelium by processes which are similar to those that have been described in a variety of other absorptive and secretory epithelital cells, e.g. in the gut (see Chapters 4 and 5).

On the basolateral membrane of the epithelial cell, a Na^+,K^+-ATPase pump is responsible for active transport of Na^+. On the luminal membrane, there are Cl^- and Na^+ channels, both of which are driven by passive processes (Fig. 5).

Because of these transport systems, the airway surface epithelium exhibits the ability

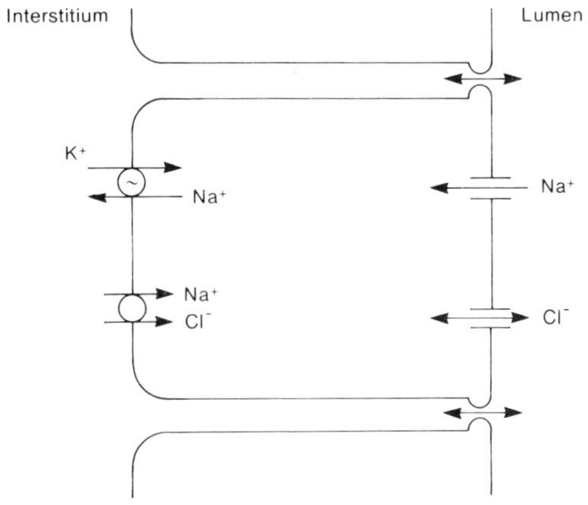

Fig. 5. Diagram of principal ion transport pathways across epithelial cells
Reprinted with permission from [12].

for both net absorption and secretion of salt and of liquid, as water passively follows the electrolytes. Under basal conditions, the surface epithelium of the large conducting airways exhibits liquid absorption, driven by active Na^+ transport. The surface epithelium also secretes liquid, driven by active Cl^- transport in the basolateral membrane. This process is stimulated by a number of substances (e.g. arachidonic acid metabolites, neuropeptides, β-adrenoceptor agonists), and the surface epithelia may therefore secrete Cl^- and water during pathological conditions [12]. Thus, the direction of the transepithelial passage of electrolytes and water is from the lumen to the submucosa under physiological conditions, but it can be reversed by inflammation. Active ion and water transport across the airway epithelium is probably of importance for hydration of mucus and for regulating the thickness of the periciliary fluid layer [13].

Epithelial synthesis of macromolecules

Recent data indicate that, in addition to the gland cells, the ciliated surface cells may contribute to the macromolecular content of the surface liquid. The ciliated cells can produce glycoconjugate macromolecules, probably proteoglycans, which are carried to the apical cell surface. The released macromolecules can be identified as a glycocalyx of about 0.3 μm in height overlying the cell surface [38]. The precise role of these epithelial macromolecules is not known, but they could possibly interact with mucin and contribute to the viscoelastic properties of the gel. As the surface cells are devoid of secretory granules, they are not classic secretory cells.

> ▶ The submucosal glands are under the control of the parasympathetic nervous system, a dense network of cholinergic nerve endings residing in these areas; neuropeptides of the NANC nervous system also stimulate gland secretion.
> ▶ Stimulation of C-fibre sensory nerves initiates an axon reflex which produces mucus secretion; C-fibres are thought to become more easily stimulated (sensitized) in airways disease.

> ▶ During inflammation, a variety of cells release biochemical mediators, such as secretagogues which stimulate mucus production; in addition, the direction of the transepithelial passage of water and ions — from the lumen to the submucosa — may be reversed.

Diseases

A variety of airways diseases, including rhinitis, asthma, chronic bronchitis and cystic fibrosis, are associated, at least intermittently, with excessive production of respiratory secretions.

Allergic and non-allergic rhinitis

Allergen challenge of a sensitized nasal mucosa results in profuse watery rhinorrhea within minutes. The major part of the liquid is believed to be a reflex-mediated glandular product, as pretreatment by atropine markedly reduces the response [39, 40]. In addition, unilateral provocation is followed by contralateral discharge, indicating reflex-activation of glands [41]. Increased albumin levels indicate that there is also a contribution from plasma exudation [33]. The role played by axon reflexes and by direct glandular effect of inflammatory secretagogues is unknown, and probably small.

In non-allergic or vasomotor rhinitis, the amount of watery rhinorrhea can be reduced by about 40% by treatment with a spray containing the cholinergic receptor antagonist, ipratropium bromide. Thus, at least 40% of the nasal discharge is a reflex-mediated glandular product. Cold air-induced rhinorrhea can be reduced by 70% with the same treatment [42].

Common cold

The watery rhinorrhea during the first days of a cold is also mediated, in part, via glandular cholinoceptors, as it can be 50% reduced by treatment with ipratropium bromide [42]. This treatment, however, has little or no effect on the viscous purulent discharge, which is probably composed of glandular mucus released by inflammatory secretagogues, plasma exudation and cellular debris (including DNA).

Virus-induced sloughing of ciliated cells and reduced mucociliary transport can also contribute to nasal discharge and sputum production in viral airway infections [43].

Otitis media

Middle ear diseases are mentioned briefly because the middle ear is lined with a ciliated epithelium, similar to the airway epithelium, and it is easy to sample secretions. Thus, otitis media can serve as a model disease for various types of discharge.

Examples of conditions caused by plasma transudation/exudation are barotrauma and acute serous otitis media. The fluid is yellow with a high concentration of albumin and other plasma proteins. It has the physical characteristics of plasma and it is not a viscoelastic gel.

Secretory otitis media provides us with an example of secretion from mucous cells. There is an increased number of goblet cells and a new formation of abnormal submucosal glands (there are no glands in the normal middle ear) [14]. The secretion in secretory otitis media is a colourless gel which is extremely viscous.

In chronic infectious otitis media, there is a similar hyperplasia of mucous cells, as in secretory otitis media, but there is also a considerable admixture of DNA from dead neutrophils, which colours the secretion and gives it a relatively high viscosity and low elasticity.

The discharge in acute infectious otitis media is composed of mucus from goblet cells, plasma exudation and cellular debris.

Sinusitis

There is no coherent gland layer in the paranasal sinuses. In the maxillary sinus, there are only approximately 50 small glands around the ostium [14]. Consequently, the mucus in acute sinusitis is predominantly a goblet cell product with admixture of cellular debris (including DNA). In chronic sinusitis, however, new submucosal glands develop. They are not innervated, are morphologically abnormal and may undergo cystic degeneration.

Asthma

Although asthma in non-smokers is not associated with daily sputum production, mucus plays an important role in this condition. An asthma attack is usually terminated by the expectoration of a small amount of very viscous mucus, and patients who die from asthma have their peripheral airways plugged by mucus containing eosinophils and desquamated epithelial cells.

Strictly speaking, we do not know whether the mucus plugging of the airways is caused by an excess of normal secretion, an abnormal secretion including plasma exudate, or simply by the entrapment of normal volumes of normal secretions by intense bronchoconstriction. It is likely that increased mucus production, plasma exudation, abnormal viscoelastic properties and impaired clearance all contribute to the abnormalities observed.

Mast cell activation, which is assumed to be central to asthma, results in the release of mediators which, as inflammatory secretagogues, may stimulate glands directly, as well as indirectly by both CNS and axon reflexes. In addition, plasma exudation will expose airway secretory cells to plasma secretagogues, and the leakage of plasma proteins will add to both volume and viscosity of the airway surface liquid (Table 1).

The inflammation in asthma is characterized by massive infiltration of eosinophils which, upon activation, release cytotoxic peptides [44]. This may contribute to the epithelial shedding in the constricted airways and may result in impaired mucociliary transport. Retention of mucus within the airways and shearing as a result of bronchial smooth muscle contraction will contribute to the high viscosity of mucus. Experimental studies have shown that mild shearing of mucus followed by stasis causes an 80-fold increase in viscosity at low shear rates — a situation which may be present in asthma [45].

Plasma exudation can be controlled effectively by the administration of steroids. Thus, the pronounced effect of steroid treatment on all asthma symptoms, including 'hypersecretion' suggests that plasma exudation plays a role in this condition [35, 36]. However, only secreted mucus, and not exuded plasma, can account for the viscoelastic properties of the mucous plugs in the asthmatic airways.

Atropine and ipratropium bromide act as bronchodilators, but, apparently, they have no effect on the amount and viscoelasticity of sputum in asthma [2, 17]. This indicates that reflex-activation of glands does not play an important role in asthma. It is difficult to explain why there should be such a marked difference between upper airways (rhinitis) and lower airways (asthma).

Chronic bronchitis

Chronic bronchitis is characterized by sputum production, recurrent infections and airway

Table 1 **Possible causes of mucus impaction in asthma**

Glandular hypersecretion
parasympathetic reflex
axon reflex
inflammatory secretagogues
Plasma exudation
inflammatory mediators
Increased mucus viscosity
impaired mucus flow due to bronchoconstriction
plasma proteins
DNA from dead eosinophils and epithelial cells
Reduced clearance
damage of cilia and epithelium
from eosinophil substances
from sticky mucus
from squeezing

obstruction. In most cases, it is caused by tobacco smoking.

Tobacco smoke has a series of effects which can all lead to acute discharge of mucus:

— (i) it stimulates nervous C-fibre receptors to release SP
— (ii) it increases the permeability of surface epithelium and of blood vessels
— (iii) it recruits neutrophils to the mucous membrane
— (iv) it stimulates surface goblet cells directly.

Smoking also has a chronic effect on the mucous membrane. Rats exposed to cigarette smoke, or to SO_2, develop significant goblet cell and submucosal gland hyperplasia [15, 46], and the same is the case for humans who volunteer for long-term exposure to tobacco smoke. Thus, the daily stimulation of the glands and goblet cells may, in the long run, result in hyperplasia [47].

Contributing to sputum production are a reduced number of ciliated cells and impaired mucociliary clearance. Stagnation of mucus in the airways predisposes to bacterial infections which further increase mucus production and decrease ciliary activity.

Atropine slows down mucociliary clearance and decreases sputum weight by a moderate amount, while inhaled ipratropium bromide apparently is devoid of these effects [48]. Steroid treatment has no significant effect on sputum production in chronic bronchitis. Thus, neither reflex-mediated glandular hypersecretion nor plasma exudation seems to be important for the volume of sputum in chronic bronchitis.

Cystic fibrosis

Patients with cystic fibrosis have a genetic defect of the protein controlling the Cl^- channels, which become less permeable [12]. An abnormal salt and water transport over the airway epithelium probably results in a reduced periciliary fluid layer and, consequently, impaired mucociliary clearance. There is a predilection for infections and, with time, the airway lumen becomes filled with tenacious and thick mucus, the lung function is impaired, and untreated patients die at a young age. (See Chapters 4 and 5.)

Primary ciliary dyskinesia

At the beginning of this century, Kartagener [49] described a triad consisting of chronic rhinosinusitis, chronic bronchitis with bronchiectases, and situs inversus. A decade ago it was shown that this syndrome is caused by an inborn defect in cilia, which causes them to beat in an unco-ordinated way, so that mucociliary clearance is zero [50]. This disease is now called primary ciliary dyskinesia or 'the immotile cilia syndrome', which is a misnomer as most patients have motile cilia.

Patients with primary ciliary dyskinesia clear the secretions from the nose by blowing, and from the tracheobronchial airways by coughing. For aerodynamic reasons, it is not possible to clear the small airways by cough (see Chapter 10). Nevertheless these patients do not suffer from mucus plugging of the peripheral airways. It is difficult to explain why they, in contrast to untreated cystic fibrosis patients, can survive for decades. Properly treated, they can live a long life.

Primary ciliary dyskinesia serves as a model disease to show the physiological significance of mucociliary transport, and we must conclude that ciliary activity seems to be less important than had been thought earlier.

► A variety of airways diseases are associated with excessive production of respiratory secretions, with marked differences between upper airways infections and lower airways infections.
► The mucus of rhinorrhea is composed mainly of a reflex-mediated glandular product; by comparison, plasma exudation is thought to be more important in asthma.
► The daily stimulation of glands and goblet cells by the irritants in tobacco can result in the hyperplasia associated with chronic bronchitis.
► Primary ciliary dyskinesia results from an inborn defect in cilia, which causes them to beat in an unco-ordinated way that prevents mucociliary clearance.

References

1. Kaliner, M., Marom, Z., Patow, C. and Shelhamer, J. (1984) Human respiratory mucus. J. Allergy Clin. Immunol. **73**, 318–323.
2. Kaliner, M. A., Shelhamer, J. H., Borson, D. J., Nadel, J. A., Patow, C. A. and Marom, Z. (1988) Respiratory mucus. In The Airways. Neural Control in Health and Disease (Kaliner, M. A. and Barnes, P. J., eds.), pp. 575–599, Marcel Dekker Inc., New York
3. Brofeldt, S., Mygind, N., Sørensen, C. H., Readman, A. S. and Marriott, C. (1986) Biochemical analysis of nasal secretions induced by methalcholine, histamine, and allergen provocations. Am. Rev. Respir. Dis. **133**, 1138–1142
4. Richardson, P. S. and Phipps, R. J. (1978) The anatomy, physiology, pharmacology and pathology of tracheobronchial mucus secretion and use of expectorant drugs in human disease. Pharmacol. Therapeut. B **3**, 441–479
5. Basbaum, C. B. and Finkbeiner, W. E. (1988) Mucus-producing cells of the airways. In Lung Cell Biology (Massaro, D., ed.), pp. 37–79, Marcel Dekker Inc., New York
6. Brofeldt, S. and Mygind, N. (1987) Viscosity and spinability of nasal secretions induced by different provocation tests. Am. Rev. Respir. Dis. **136**, 353–356
7. Toremalm, N.-G. (1960) The daily amount of tracheobronchial secretions in man. Acta Otolaryngol. (Stockholm) **158** (Suppl.), 43
8. Ueki, I., German, V. F. and Nadel, J. A. (1980) Micropipette measurement of airway submucosal gland secretion. Autonomic effects. Am. Rev. Respir. Dis. **121**, 351–357
9. Mygind, N. and Thomsen, J. (1976) Diurnal variation of nasal protein concentration. Acta Otolaryngol. (Stockholm) **82**, 219–221
10. Bateman, J. R. M., Pavia, D. and Clarke, S. W. (1978) The retention of lung secretions during the night in normal subjects. Clin. Sci. **55**, 523
11. Lucas, A. M. and Douglas, L. C. (1934) Principles underlying ciliary activity in the respiratory tract. Arch. Otolaryngol. **20**, 518–541
12. Knowles, M. R., Fisher, S., Kenan, P., Pillsbury, H. C. and Brofeldt, S. (1987) Nasal secretions: role of epithelial ion transport. In Allergic and Vasomotor Rhinitis: Pathophysiological Aspects (Mygind, N. and Pipkorn, U., eds.), pp. 77–90, Munksgaard, Copenhagen
13. Frizzell, R. A. (1988) Role of absorptive and secretory processes in hydration of the airway surface. Am. Rev. Respir. Dis. **138**, S3–S6
14. Tos, M. (1983) Distribution of mucus producing elements in the respiratory tract. Differences between upper and lower airways. Eur. J. Respir. Dis. **64** (Suppl. **128**), 269–279
15. Reid, L. (1963) An experimental study of hypersecretion of mucus in the bronchial tree. Thorax **44**, 437–445
16. Cauna, H., Hinderer, K. H., Manzetti, G. W. and Swanson, E. W. (1972) Fine structure of nasal polyps. Ann. Otol. Rhinol. Laryngol. **81**, 41–48
17. Lundgren, J. D. and Shelhamer, J. H. (1990) Pathogenesis of airway mucus hypersecretion. J. Allergy Clin. Immunol. **85**, 399–417
18. Takizawa, T. and Thurlbeck, W. M. (1971) Muscle and mucous gland size in the major bronchi of patients with chronic bronchitis, asthma, and asthmatic bronchitis. Am. Rev. Respir. Dis. **104**, 331–336
19. Tos, M. (1981) Goblet cells and glands in the nose and paranasal sinuses. In The Nose: Upper Airway Physiology and the Atmospheric Environment (Andersen, I. and Proctor, D. F., eds.), pp. 99–144, Elsevier Biomedical Press, Amsterdam
20. Lopez-Vidriero, M. T., Das, I., Smith, A. P., Picot, R. and Reid, L. (1977) Bronchial secretion from normal human airways after inhalation of prostaglandin F2alpha, acetylcholine, histamine and citric acid. Thorax **32**, 734–739
21. Murlas, C., Nadel, J. A. and Basbaum, C. B. (1980) A morphometric analysis of the autonomic innervation of cat tracheal glands. J. Autonomic Nerv. Syst. **2**, 23–37
22. Borum, P. (1979) Nasal methacholine challenge. A test for the measurement of nasal reactivity. J. Allergy Clin. Immunol. **63**, 253–257
23. Basbaum, C. B., Ueki, I., Brezina, L. and Nadel, J. A. (1981) Tracheal submucosal gland serous cells stimulated *in vitro* with adrenergic and cholinergic agonists: a morphometric study. Cell Tissue Res. **220**, 481–498
24. Leikauf, G. D., Ueki, I. F. and Nadel, J. A. (1984) Autonomic regulation of viscoelasticity of cat tracheal gland secretions. J. Appl. Physiol. **56**, 426–430
25. Borson, D. B. and Nadel, J. A. (1990) Regulation of airway secretions: role of peptides and proteases. In Rhinitis and Asthma: Similarities and Differences (Mygind, N., Pipkorn, U. and Dahl, R., eds.), pp. 76–99, Munksgaard, Copenhagen
26. Gashi, A. A., Borson, D. B., Finkbeiner, W. E., Nadel, J. A. and Basbaum, C. B. (1986) Neuropeptides degranulate serous cells of ferret tracheal glands. Am. J. Physiol. **251**(20), C223–C229
27. Shimura, A., Sasaki, T., Okayama, H. and Takishima, T. (1987) The effect of substance P on mucus secretion of isolated submucosal gland from feline trachea. J. Appl. Physiol. **63**, 646–653
28. Lundblad, L. (1990) Neuropeptides and autonomic nervous control of the respiratory mucosa. In Rhinitis and Asthma: Similarities and Differences (Mygind, N.,

Pipkorn, U. and Dahl, R., eds.), pp. 65–75, Munksgaard, Copenhagen
29. Barnes, P. (1986) Asthma as an axon reflex. Lancet 1, 242
30. Stjarne, P., Lundblad, L., Lundberg, J. M. and Anggård, A. (1989) Capsaicin and nicotine-sensitive afferent neurones and nasal secretion in healthy human volunteers and in patients with vasomotor rhinitis. Br. J. Pharmacol. 96, 693–701
31. Hunter, J. A., Finkbeiner, W. E., Nadel, J. A., Goetzl, E. J. and Holtzman, M. J. (1985) Predominant generation of 15-lipoxygenase metabolites of arachidonic acid by epithelial cells from human trachea. Proc. Natl. Acad. Sci. U.S.A. 82, 4633–4637
32. Jones, R. and Reid, L. (1978) Secretory cell hyperplasia and modification of intracellular glycoprotein in rat airways induced by short periods of exposure to tobacco smoke, and the effect of the antiinflammatory agent phenylmethyloxadiazole. Lab. Invest. 39, 41–49
33. Pipkorn, U., Proud, D., Lichtenstein, L. M., Schleimer, R. P., Peters, S. P., Adkinson, Jr N. F., Kagey-Sobotka, A., Norman, P. S. and Naclerio, R. M. (1987) Effect of short-term systemic glucocorticoid treatment on human nasal mediator release after antigen challenge. J. Clin. Invest. 80, 957–961
34. Svensson, C., Baumgarten, C. R., Pipkorn, U., Alkner, U. and Persson, C. G. A. (1989) Reversibility and reproducibility of histamine induced plasma leakage in nasal airways. Thorax 44, 13–18
35. Persson, C. G. A. and Erjefalt, I. (1988) Nonneural and neural regulation of plasma exudation in airways. In The Airways: Neural Control in Health and Disease (Kaliner, M. A. and Barnes, P. J., eds.), pp. 523–549, Marcel Dekker Inc., New York
36. Persson, C. G. A. (1986) Role of plasma exudation in asthmatic airways. Lancet ii, 1126–1129
37. Persson, C. G. A. and Pipkorn, U. (1990) Pathogenesis and pharmacology of asthma and rhinitis. In Rhinitis and Asthma: Similarities and Differences (Mygind, N., Pipkorn, U. and Dahl, R., eds.), pp. 275–288, Munksgaard, Copenhagen
38. Varsano, S., Basbaum, C. B., Forsberg, L. S., Borson, D. B., Caughey, G. and Nadel, J. A. (1987) Dog tracheal epithelial cells in culture synthesize sulfated macromolecular glycoconjugates and release them from the cell surface upon exposure to extracellular proteinases. Exp. Lung Res. 13, 157–183
39. Konno, A., Togawa, K. and Fujiwara, T. (1983) The mechanisms involved in onset of allergic manifestations in the nose. Eur. J. Respir. Dis. 64 (Suppl. 128), 155–166
40. Konno, A., Terada, N., Okamoto, Y. and Togawa, K. (1987) The role of chemical mediators and mucosal hyperreactivity in nasal hypersecretion in nasal allergy. J. Allergy Clin. Immunol. 79, 620–626
41. Okuda, M. (1977) Mechanisms in nasal allergy. ORL Digest 39, 22–26
42. Mygind, N. and Borum, P. (1990) Anticholinergic treatment of watery rhinorrhea. Am. J. Rhinol. 4, 1–5
43. Pedersen, M., Sakakura, Y., Winther, B., Brofeldt, S. and Mygind, N. (1983) Nasal mucociliary transport, number of ciliated cells, and beating pattern in naturally acquired common cold. Eur. J. Respir. Dis. 64 (Suppl. 128), 355–365
44. Venge, P., Dahl, R., Fredens, K. and Peterson, C. G. B. (1988) Epithelial injury by human eosinophils. Am. Rev. Respir. Dis. 138, S54–S57
45. Sturgess, J., Palfrey, A. J. and Reid, L. (1971) Rheological properties of sputum. Rheology Acta 10, 36–43
46. Mawdesley-Thomas, L. E., Healey, P. and Barry, D. H. (1971) Experimental bronchitis in animals due to sulphur dioxide and animal smoke. An automated quantitative study. In Inhaled Particles III (Walton, W. H., ed.), pp. 509–525, The Gresham Press, Surrey
47. Thurlbeck, W. M. (1977) Aspects of chronic airflow obstruction. Chest 72, 341–349
48. Hahn, H.-L. (1988) Anticholinergic drugs in bronchial asthma. In The Airways: Neural Control in Health and Disease (Kaliner, M. A. and Barnes, P. J., eds.), pp. 241–279, Marcel Dekker Inc., New York
49. Kartagener, M. (1933) Zur pathogenese der Bronkietasien bei situs viscerum inversus. Beitr. Klin. Tuberk. 83, 489–501
50. Mygind, N., Nielsen, M. H. and Pedersen, M. (eds.) (1983) Kartagener's syndrome and abnormal cilia. Eur. J. Respir. Dis. 64 (Suppl. 127), 1–167
51. Satir, P. (1974) How cilia move. Sci. Am. 231, 45
52. Proetz, A. W. (1953) Applied Physiology of the Nose, Annals Publishing Company, St Louis

7

Diarrhoea and intestinal hypersecretion

N. W. Read
Centre for Human Nutrition, Northern General Hospital, Herries Road, Sheffield S5 7AN, U.K.

Introduction

Under normal circumstances the gastro-intestinal tract is adapted for the digestion and absorption of nutrients, but, when the gut is inflamed or invaded by noxious organisms or toxins, its functions are co-ordinated to clear the gut of its contents. Clearance of the gut involves vomiting and diarrhoea. Thus, diarrhoea may be seen as one component of a protective mechanism. For efficient clearance to take place, it must involve both epithelial secretion of fluid and propulsion of gastro-intestinal contents. This review is concerned primarily with the mechanism of hypersecretion in diarrhoea, but it is impossible to consider this without making comparisons with the mechanism underlying gastro-intestinal propulsion and discussing the inter-relationship between the two processes.

The cellular mechanism of intestinal absorption and secretion

The absorption of fluid across the intestinal epithelium is thought to be generated by the osmotic gradients produced in the lateral intercellular space, and possibly also the sub-epithelial space, by the transport of solute. In the most accepted mechanism, sodium is transported across the microvillous membrane by facilitated diffusion, either by itself or in association with other solutes such as sugars, amino acids, chloride and, in the colon, short-chain fatty acids [1]. The diffusion gradient for sodium powers the entry of the co-transported solutes into the cell. Sodium is then actively transported across the serosal membrane into the lateral space by means of a specific sodium- and potassium-dependent ATPase, while the co-transported solutes exit into the same space by facilitated diffusion. The increase in lateral space osmolality then encourages the flow of water in from the lumen, expanding the lateral space and causing fluid to flow along the line of least resistance to the subepithelial capillaries. This inwardly directed flow of water may be facilitated by a substrate-dependent increase in tight junction permeability [2].

Secretion of fluid into the intestine lumen can take place when hyperosmotic solutions enter the lumen or in response to increases in epithelial permeability, but secretion induced by bacterial toxins, or the release of neurotransmitters, hormones or autacoids, is thought to occur as a consequence of active transcellular ion secretion from the enterocytes. Until recently, active secretion was thought to take place largely in the crypts between the villi of the small intestine and in the colonic crypts. It now appears, however, that all enterocytes possess the capacity to secrete fluid, but, as cells mature and climb the villous escalator, they acquire the machinery for absorption. The ionic basis of active intestinal secretion is an increase in chloride permeability at the lumen membrane [1]. As chloride diffuses out of the cell, the transfer of negative charge causes the epithelial surface to become more negative which encourages the flow of sodium through the tight junctions into the lumen. Water follows the serosa to mucosa flow of ions by osmosis (Fig. 1). Other processes, such as capillary dilatation, an increase in capillary permeability and perhaps a change in the configuration of the tight junctions, are likely to take place at the same time to facilitate secretion.

Secretion can be induced by the interaction of transmitter substances with receptors on the cell surface. These set in motion a sequence of

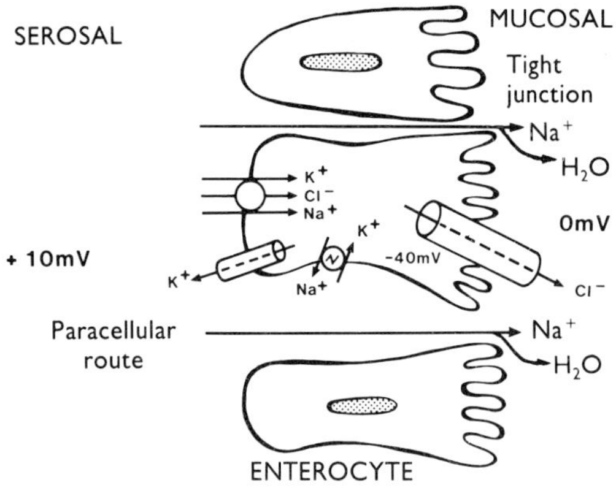

Fig. 1. The ion transport mechanisms that subserve active intestinal secretion

events [3] which involve the turnover of phosphatidylinositol and an increase in cytosolic calcium, and/or catalyse the formation of cyclic nucleotides. Both cyclic nucleotides and calcium may then activate protein kinases, which in turn phosphorylate membrane proteins and alter mucosal permeability (Fig. 2).

The enteric nervous control of intestinal transport

It seems likely that both secretion and absorption are taking place all the time. Under basal conditions, when there is little glucose in the lumen and, particularly after a meal, the small intestine is in a state of net absorption. But when the epithelium is damaged, infected, or exposed to toxins or irritants, active secretion predominates. The balance between absorption and secretion — the transport tone of the intestine — is modulated by activity in the enteric nervous system [4].

Blockade of the enteric nervous system with the neurotoxin, tetrodotoxin, increases the mucosal to serosal flux of sodium and chloride ions and decreases short circuit current, suggesting that the net effect of an indiscriminate increase in activity in the enteric nervous system is to reduce absorption and enhance secretion. This conclusion is supported by depolarization of the enteric nervous system either by scorpion venom, or by passing an electrical current in the plane of the epithelium (electrical field stimulation) [5]. Both stimuli increase serosal to mucosal ion fluxes and short circuit current. These studies do not exclude the possibility that a selective stimulation of some enteric nerves, for example after activation of the sympathetic nervous system, can increase absorption and reduce short circuit current.

Studies using Ussing chambers (see Chapter 5) have identified a very large number of transmitter substances [e.g. vasoactive intestinal polypeptide (VIP), 5-hydroxytryptamine (5-HT), prostaglandin E_1, substance P, acetylcholine (ACh) and bradykinin] which can influence intestinal transport. Receptor binding studies suggest that only some of these act at the level of the enterocyte and it seems likely that most of them act on enteric neurons [4].

If activity within the enteric nervous system controls the 'transport tone' of the intestine, factors that cause diarrhoea probably act by stimulating enteric nervous reflexes which enhance intestinal secretion. Thus,

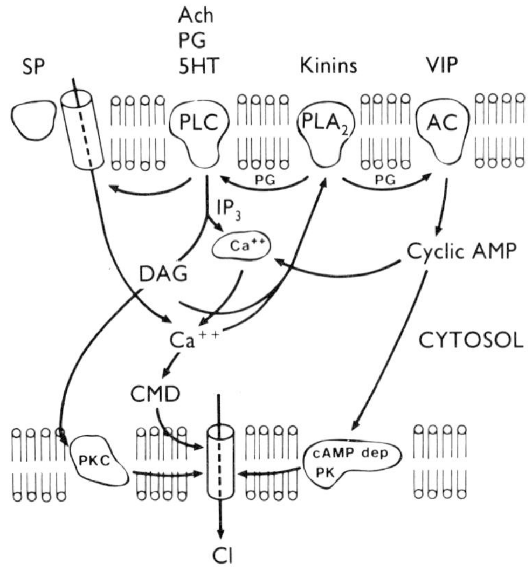

2. The intracellular mediators and their interactions in the production of active intestinal secretion

Abbreviations used: AC, adenylyl cyclase; ACh, acetylcholine; cAMP-dep PK, cyclic AMP-dependent protein kinase; CMD, calmodulin; DAG, diacylglycerol; 5HT, 5-hydroxytryptamine; IP₃, inositol triphosphate; PG, prostaglandin; PKC, protein kinase C; PLA₂, phospholipase A₂; PLC, phospholipase C; SP, substance P; VIP, vasoactive intestinal polypeptide.

diarrhoea may perhaps be considered to be an 'enteric nervous disorder'.

Enteric reflexes

One of the first indications of involvement of enteric nervous reflexes in the pathogenesis of diarrhoea was the discovery by Lundgren's group that the secretion associated with cholera in the cat could be suppressed by tetrodotoxin, ganglion blockers and local anaesthetics, and was associated with the release of VIP, a potent secretagogue, from nerve endings into the blood draining the gut [6]. Similar experiments carried out by the same group indicate that other enterotoxins, laxatives and bile acids, as well as prostaglandins and arachidonic acid, when administered into the lumen to induce inflammatory states [6], may also induce secretion by stimulating enteric reflexes. Other investigators using Ussing chambers were unable to show that tetrodotoxin had any effect on cholera-induced electrolyte secretion [7, 8], but it is possible that the reflex secretion was mediated via long nerve loops that were damaged during preparation of the biopsies. The current view is that cholera-toxin induces intestinal secretion both by a direct action on enterocytes and by triggering enteric reflexes, but the relative contribution of each is uncertain.

Evidence suggests that mechanical stimulation of the muscosa can also induce motility changes [9] and secretion via enteric reflexes. The secretion that is stimulated by stroking the epithelium with a glass rod or by distension of the gut can be blocked by ganglion blockers and local anaesthetics [10].

Secretion may also be elicited by contractile activity in the gut. We showed some years ago that certain types of propagated contractions were associated with pronounced elevations of the transmural potential difference (PD) indicating a change in intestinal transport [11]. These elevations were not mechanical artefacts because they peaked about 45 s *after* the pressure events. Similar increases in PD were induced by distension of the gut, and blocked by hexamethonium. Luminal distension releases neurotransmitters such as ACh, 5-HT and prostaglandins, all of which induce intestinal secretion and elevate the PD. These data (for review, see [12]) suggest that rises in PD related to contractile events may represent bursts of intestinal secretion. The most compelling argument in favour of this concept, however, is the observation that patients with cystic fibrosis, who lack the chloride carrier, show no increases in PD, either in response to secretagogues or in association with bursts of motor activity [13] (see Chapter 5).

► Diarrhoea is a protective mechanism which clears the intestine of its contents when it becomes distended or invaded by noxious organisms or toxins; it is brought about by a combination of hypersecretion and gastro-intestinal propulsion.
► Factors that cause diarrhoea probably act by stimulating enteric nervous reflexes to reduce absorption and enhance secretion.
► Transmitter substances, e.g. 5-HT and VIP, enhance intestinal secretion; most act on enteric nerves while a few act directly on the enterocyte.
► Mechanical stimulation of the mucosa or contractile activity of the gut may also induce intestinal secretion.

Role of 5-HT and autacoids

The hypersecretion induced by cholera-toxin can be blocked or severely inhibited by 5-HT receptor antagonists or 5-HT tachyphylaxis [14]. This suggests a fairly crucial role for 5-HT in mediating or enhancing the secretory response. 5-HT can be released from enterochromaffin cells in the epithelium. Cytofluorometric studies have shown a reduction in the 5-HT content of enterochromaffin cells after exposure to cholera-toxin [6]. 5-HT, presumably released from enterochromaffin cells, is thought to activate afferent nerve endings [6]. It is probable, however, that other entero-endocrine cells, releasing other transmitters, can be degranulated by luminal stimuli that induce secretion [15]. Cholera-toxin-induced secretion can also be abolished by indomethacin and restored by administration of prostaglandin PGE_1 [6]. 5-HT is also located in a sub-population of enteric neurons and can be released by stimuli activating these neurons. It has a role as a neuromodulator and neurotransmitter in the enteric nervous system.

Damage to the epithelium can release various substances such as prostaglandins, bradykinins, histamine and 5-HT, which mediate components of the inflammatory response and cause secretion [4]. This presumably serves to dilute toxic or damaging substances in the lumen. The effect of luminal prostaglandins can be blocked by tetrodotoxin [6], suggesting that inflammatory mediators may induce secretion via an enteric nervous loop.

Mast cells may play a crucial role in certain types of secretory response. They can be degranulated during irritation or damage to the epithelium, as well as by the specific combination of antigen with immunoglobulin E antibodies. Proliferation of submucosal mast cells is a feature of food allergy, coeliac disease, parasitic infestations, some patients with Irritable Bowel Syndrome (IBS), inflammatory bowel disease and other conditions associated with diarrhoea [16]. Mast cells release a whole cocktail of transmitter substances, many of which can induce intestinal secretion. They tend to accumulate around enteric nerves [17] and form quite intimate connections with them. This suggests the possibility of not only degranulation of mast cells by activity in nerves, but also the subsequent activation of enteric nervous system elements by this process (Fig. 3).

Sensitization of enteric reflexes

It seems likely that in many instances diarrhoea may result from enhancement or sensitization of enteric reflexes. Three examples are given below.

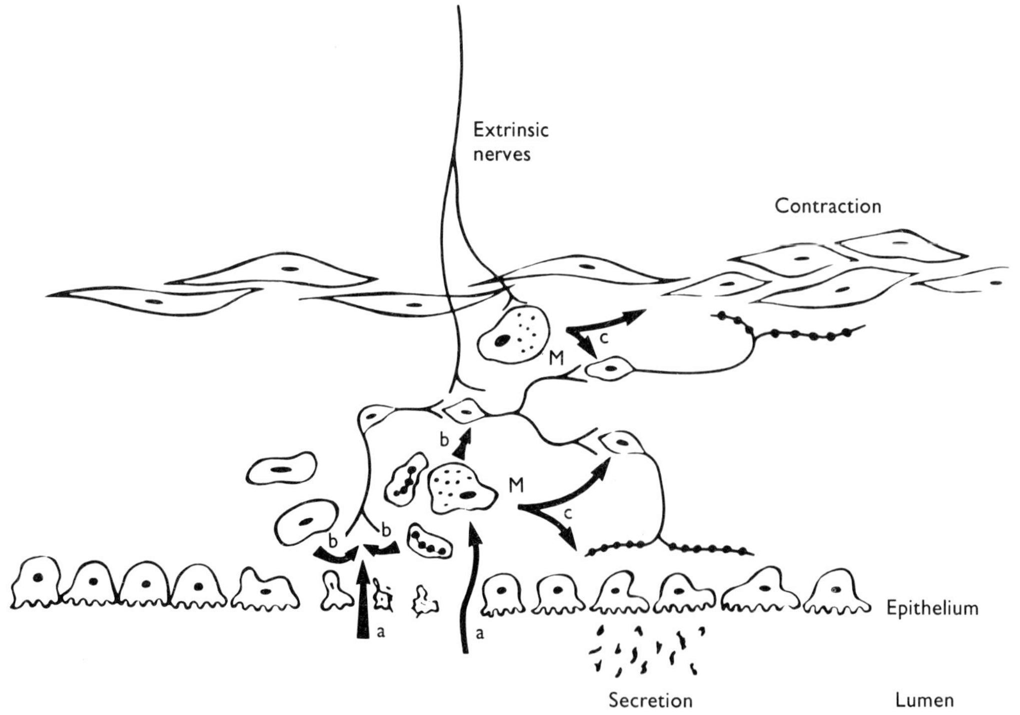

Fig. 3. Interactions between the immune system and the enteric nervous system to cause intestinal secretion and propulsive motility

*Arrows '**a**' show the release of mediators from damaged cells to interact with mast cells (M) and enteric nerve terminals. Arrows '**b**' show the release of transmitters from inflammatory cells and mast cells to interact with afferent nerve terminals and enteric ganglia. Arrows '**c**' indicate how mast cell products directly cause secretion and motor changes.*

Immunological sensitization

Immunological sensitization of the gut to specific antigens can result in intestinal hypersecretion, and in an increase in short circuit current and PD when the gut is further exposed to that antigen. Sensitization can be induced in experimental animals by substituting drinking water for milk, by parasitic infestation, by intraperitoneal injections and by damaging the epithelium with bile acids, detergents and u.v. light [18, 19]. The mediators of this effect differ in different species, but experiments using specific inhibitors have implicated histamine, 5-HT, prostaglandins and tachykinins. These experiments would offer an explanation for reports of IBS following an attack of gastro-enteritis, and for a type of food-related diarrhoea [20]. It is possible that damage to the mucosa by enteric pathogens may allow access of protein antigens to the sub-epithelial space where they may sensitize mast cells.

Recent evidence suggests that these reflexes may be conditioned in the rat. Bienenstock [21] has shown that, if a bell is rung every time that food containing the antigen is administered, then after a time the bell itself induces degranulation of mast cells. This suggests that nerves may be able to make connections with sensitized immunoreactive elements. Indeed, degranulation of mast cells is highly chemoattractant to enteric nerves.

Starvation

Somewhat surprisingly, diarrhoea is a severe and often terminal complication of starvation or malnutrition. It is commonly thought to be related to vitamin deficiency or opportunist infection with enteric pathogens. However, there is new evidence to suggest that starvation may sensitize the epithelium to secretagogues. Young and Levin [22] have shown that, after rats have been starved for three days, the intestine secretes much more fluid and generates a much higher short circuit current in response to a variety of secretagogues. The observations that (i) some of these agents, bethanecol for example, act directly on the secretory enterocyte, and that (ii) hypersecretion occurs only in response to those transmitters that act by gating calcium, and not in response to agents that act by increasing the concentration of cyclic nucleotides, suggests that this phenomenon is related to a change in cellular response to transmitters rather than an activation of enteric reflexes. Chronic food deprivation, caused by giving rats only 33% of their normal energy supplies, causes a much more prolonged hypersecretion than complete starvation. Discovery of the factors that mediate this adaptive response could help to prevent a major cause of morbidity and mortality in the 'developing world'.

Irritable Bowel Syndrome

A major sub-set of patients with IBS have an increase in rectal sensitivity and motor reactivity of the gut in response to stimuli such as distension, food, stress and injections of cholecystokinin. Most attention has been paid to motor phenomena in IBS, but it seems likely that there is a comparative sensitization of transport tone. Many patients with IBS complain of diarrhoea. At proctoscopy, there is often abundant mucus in some patients with IBS. Oddson et al. [23] produced the only scientific evidence of hypersecretion in IBS by demonstrating that the secretory response of the ileum to the bile acid, glycochenodeoxycholic acid, was enhanced in such patients. They suggest that this increased response might be related to release of prostaglandins.

The relationship between motility and secretion

Clearance of the gut involves both secretion and propulsive motor activity. It is therefore interesting that many of the factors that cause reflex secretion — enterotoxins, laxative agents and bile acids — also cause propulsive or propagated motor activity [12]. Studies in loops of rabbit ileum suggest these factors may act via the enteric nervous system. Mathias and his colleagues [24] have shown that these agents can induce migrating action potential complexes (MAPCs) in isolated loops of rabbit ileum, which can be blocked with tetrodotoxin and ganglion blockers. Although distension caused by secretion can induce, at least *in vivo*, propulsive motor activity, the MAPC can occur independently of secretion. Choloragen, the inactive *precursor* of cholera-toxin, for example, can induce MAPCs without causing secretion, while the motor effects induced by sennosides can occur without and before a major fluid accumulation in the intestinal lumen [25]. Whether MAPCs seen in loops of rabbit ileum are an appropriate model for propulsive contractile activity seen in man is a subject of some controversy. Cowles and Sarna [26], for example, did not demonstrate an increase in propulsive motor activity in the small intestine of dogs infected with cholera.

Action of extrinsic nerves

Parasympathetic efferent fibres originating in the dorsal motor nucleus of the vagus (small intestine) or the sacral spinal cord (large intestine) synapse with enteric ganglion cells and thus may act to modulate enteric reflexes. In the cat, vagal stimulation induces intestinal secretion, but only after splanchnic nerves have been cut [27]. In the anaesthetized ferret, low frequency stimulation of the vagus nerve can cause intestinal secretion and propagated bursts of contractions [28]. The bursts of contractile activity are associated with fluctuations in PD with the peak of the PD change occurring some time after the motor event. Administration of atropine will block the propulsive motor action and the associated PD fluctuations and reduce, but not completely inhibit, secretion. This suggests that vagal stimulation activates parallel activity in the enterocytes and smooth muscle, but that the secretory response may be augmented by bursts of activity induced by contractions. In man, indirect vagal stimulation by 'sham' feeding [29] always increased gastric acid secretion, but only occasionally induced intestinal secretion.

The presence of sympathetic fibres subjacent to villous epithelial cells and the existence of adrenoreceptors on enterocytes suggests that sympathetic nerves can influence transport directly. Most adrenergic fibres, however, terminate in the submucous nerve plexus where catecholamines act on neuronal receptors to alter transport. Stimulation of the perivascular sympathetic nerves enhances absorption, reduces secretion, reduces PD and short circuit current and suppresses intestinal motor activity [27, 30].

Treatment of diarrhoea

If our implications are correct — i.e. diarrhoea is best regarded as an enteric nervous disorder — then the most effective anti-diarrhoeal agents would be those that interrupt these nervous loops without affecting the basal motor or transport function of the gut.

Opiate-like compounds are the most widely used and effective anti-diarrhoeal agents. Opiates inhibit propagated motor activity and suppress epithelial secretion. Opiate receptors have not been demonstrated on enterocytes, however, and the evidence suggests that these agents act at the level of the enteric nervous system to inhibit the release of ACh and VIP from post-ganglionic nerve terminals [31]. If this hypothesis is correct, it would explain why loperamide, a gut-selective opiate-like anti-diarrhoeal agent, fails to inhibit intestinal secretion induced by VIP [32] which acts directly on the enterocyte, but will inhibit secretion and diarrhoea induced by bile acids [33].

Diarrhoea — a unifying concept

We propose that much diarrhoeal illness may be explained on the basis of involvement of enteric nervous reflexes. There is increasing evidence that luminal stimuli, such as bile acids, bacterial enterotoxins and mucosal inflammation, may act via epithelial receptors to induce both secretion and propulsive motor activity, and that these would act together to clear the gut of its contents. In hyper-reactive states, such as the Irritable Bowel Syndrome, the gut may be sensitized to the presence of normal contents. Even malabsorptive states can result in stimulation of enteric reflexes, because malabsorbed fat and bile acid can induce colonic secretion and propulsive motor activity, and the distension caused by impaired fluid absorption may also have the same effect.

Thus, diarrhoea can be regarded as a vicious spiral [12]. It is postulated that the interaction of stimuli (chemical and mechanical) reflexly stimulates secretion and propulsive motor activity, accelerating transit and reducing contact of luminal contents with the epithelial surface. This causes a reduction in absorption and, together with the induced secretion, results in an increased luminal volume. The resulting distension further enhances secretion and motor activity and so on, resulting in copious diarrhoea.

▶ Upon stimulation, by e.g. toxins, enteroendocrine cells become degranulated and release various substances which enhance intestinal secretion; an example is the release of 5-HT from enterochromaffin cells.
▶ Diarrhoea may result from sensitization of enteric reflexes; e.g. starvation sensitizes the epithelium to secretagogues, and IBS patients exhibit increased rectal sensitivity.
▶ Many factors that cause reflex secretion also cause propulsive motor activity.

References

1. Armstrong, W. M. (1987) Cellular mechanisms of ion transport in the small intestine. In Physiology of the Gastrointestinal Tract, 2nd Edition (Johnson, L. R., ed.), pp. 1251–1265, Raven Press, New York
2. Pappenheimer, J. R. (1987) Physiological regulation of transepithelial impedance in the intestinal mucosa of rats and hamsters. J. Memb. Biol. 100,
3. Donowitz, M. and Welsh, M. J. (1987) Regulation of mammalian electrolyte secretion. In Physiology of the Gastrointestinal Tract, 2nd Edition (Johnson, L. R., ed.), pp. 1351–1388, Raven Press, New York
4. Cooke, H. J. (1987) Neural and humoral regulation of small intestinal electrolyte transport. In Physiology of the Gastrointestinal Tract, 2nd Edition (Johnson L. R., ed.), pp. 1307–1350, Raven Press, New York
5. Hubel, K. A. (1985) Intestinal nerves and ion transport: stimuli, reflexes and responses. Am. J. Physiol. **248**, G261–G274
6. Lundgren, O. (1988) Nervous control of intestinal transport. Baillieres Clin. Gastroenterol. **2**, 85–106
7. Moriarty, K. J., Higgs, N. B., Woodford, M. and Turnberg, L. A. (1986) Studies on neurological mechanisms in cholera toxin induced intestinal secretion. Proc. Eur. Intest. Transport Grp. Mtg. May 4–7th, 1986
8. Carey, H. V. and Cooke, H. J. (1986) Submucosal nerves and cholera toxin induced secretion in guinea pig ileum *in vitro*. Dig. Dis. Sci. **31**, 732–736
9. Smith, T. K., Bornstein, J. C. and Furness, J. B. (1991) Interactions between reflexes evoked by distension and mucosal stimulation: electrophysiological studies of guinea-pig ileum. J. Auton. Nerv. Syst. **34**, 69–76
10. Beubler, E. and Juan, H. (1978) PGE-release, blood flow and transmucosal water movement after mechanical stimulation of the rat jejunal mucosa. Naunyn-Schmeideberg's Arch. Pharmacol. **305**, 91–95
11. Read, N. W., Smallwood, R. H., Levin, R. J., Holdsworth, C. D. and Brown, B. H. (1977) Relationship between changes in intraluminal pressure and transmural potential difference in the human and canine jejunum *in vivo*. Gut **18**, 141–151
12. Read, N. W. (1986) Diarrhoea Motrice. Clin. Gastroenterol. **15**, 657–686
13. Baxter, P. S., Wilson, A. J. and Read, N. W. (1989) Abnormal jejunal potential in cystic fibrosis. Lancet **i**, 316–318
14. Cassuto, J., Jodal, M., Tuttle, R. and Lundgren, O. (1982) 5-hydroxytryptamine and cholera secretion. Scand. J. Gastroenterol. **17**, 695–703
15. Holmgren, J. (1981) Actions of cholera toxin and the prevention and treatment of cholera. Nature (London) **292**, 413–417
16. Miner, P. B. (1991) Systemic mastocytosis and regional gastrointestinal mast cell disease. In Irritable Bowel Syndrome (Read, N. W., ed.), pp. 174–189, Blackwell, Oxford
17. Stead, R. H., Tomioko, M., Quinonez, G., Suman, G. T., Melten, S. Y. and Bienenstock, J. (1987) Intestinal mucosal mast cells in normal and nematode infected rat intestines are in intimate contact with peptidergenic nerves. Proc. Natl. Acad. Sci. U.S.A. **84**, 2975–2979
18. Baird, A. W. and Cuthbert, A. W. (1987) Neuronal involvement in Type 1 hypersensitivity reactions in gut epithelium. Br. J. Pharmacol. **92**, 647
19. Scott, R. B., Diamant, S. C. and Gall, D. G. (1988) Motility effects of anaphylaxis in the rat. Am. J. Physiol. **255**, G505–G511
20. Alun Jones, V., Shorthouse, M., McLaughlin, P., Workman, E. and Hunter, J. O. (1982) Food intolerance: a major factor in the pathogenesis of irritable bowel syndrome. Lancet **ii**, 1115–1117
21. Bienenstock, J. (1988) An update on mast cell heterogeneity including comments on mast cell nerve relationships. J. Allerg. Clin. Immunol. **81**, 763–769
22. Young, A. and Levin, R. J. (1990) Diarrhoea of famine and malnutrition: investigations using a rat model. Jejunal hypersecretion induced by starvation. Gut **31**, 43–53
23. Oddson, E., Rask-Madsen, J. and Krag, E. (1978) A secretory epithelium of the small intestine with increased sensitivity to bile salts in IBS associated with diarrhoea. Scand. J. Gastroenterol. **13**, 409–416
24. Mathias, J. R., Carlson, G. M., Di Marino, A. J., Bertiger, G., Morton, H. E. and Cohen, S. (1976) Intestinal myoelectrical activity in response to live vibrio cholerae and cholera enterotoxin. J. Clin. Invest. **58**, 91–96
25. Leng-Peshlow, E. (1986) Dual effect of orally administered sennosides on large intestine transit and fluid absorption in the rat. J. Pharm. Pharmacol. **38**, 606–610
26. Cowles, V. E. and Sarna, S. K. (1989) Effect of cholera toxin on small intestinal motor activity in conscious dogs. Gastroenterology **94**, A912
27. Sjovall, H., Brunsson, I., Jodal, M. and Lundgren, O. (1983) The effect of vagal nerve stimulation on net fluid transport in the small intestine of the rat. Acta Physiol. Scand. **117**, 351–357
28. Greenwood, B. and Read, N. W. (1986) The effect of vagal stimulation of jejunal fluid transport, transmural potential difference and intraluminal pressure in the anaesthetized ferret. Am. J. Physiol. **12**, G651–G654
29. Read, N. W., Cooper, K. and Fordtran, J. S. (1978) Effect of modified sham feeding on jejunal transport and pancreatic and biliary secretion in man. Am. J. Physiol. **234**, E417–E420
30. Greenwood, B., Remblay, L. and Dawson, J. S. (1987) Sympathetic control of motility, fluid transport and transmural potential difference in the rabbit ileum. Am. J. Physiol. **253**, G726–G729
31. Dobbins, J. W., Dharmsathaphorn, K., Racusen, L. and Binder, N. J. (1981) The effect of somatostatin and enkephalin on ion transport in the intestine. Ann. NY Acad. Sci. **372**, 594–612
32. Schiller, L. R., Santa Ana, C. A., Morawski, S. G. and Fordtran, J. S. (1984) Mechanism of antidiarrhoeal effect of loperamide. Gastroenterology **86**, 1475–1480
33. Farack, V. M. and Loeshke, K. (1984) Inhibition by loperamide of deoxycholic acid induced intestinal secretion. Naunyn Schmeideberg's Arch. Pharmacol. **325**, 286–288

8

The pathophysiology of airway inflammation and mucosal damage in asthma

S. E. Webber and D R. Corfield
Department of Physiology, St George's Hospital Medical School, Cranmer Terrace, London SW17 0RE, U.K.

Introduction

Human bronchial asthma is characterized by a widespread and variable intrathoracic airflow obstruction. The manifestation of the asthmatic response can be divided for convenience into three stages: a rapid spasmogenic phase, a late sustained phase and a chronic underlying inflammatory phase (Fig. 1). This inflammation is often associated with structural changes including epithelial damage, increased vascular permeability and mucosal oedema, increased intraluminal secretions, basement membrane thickening and the influx of inflammatory cells including mast cells, eosinophils and neutrophils. Any explanation of the pathogenesis of asthma must take into account these structural changes; however, the mechanisms responsible have not been fully elucidated. It is clear that the mechanisms are complicated with numerous interactions between mucosal tissues, inflammatory cells and inflammatory mediators. This chapter attempts to present the knowledge of the origin of these structural changes that we have acquired to date.

Inflammatory cell infiltration and mediator release

There is no doubt that the infiltration of inflammatory cells into the airway mucosa and towards the lumen, and the subsequent release of a number of mediators, are central events in the development of inflammation and mucosal damage which is such a characteristic feature of asthma [1]. What is less clear is the type of inflammatory cell or cells (mast cells, basophils, macrophages, platelets, neutrophils, eosinophils, lymphocytes) that plays the major role. It is unlikely that one cell alone is responsible for the inflammation and mucosal damage in asthma, but all these cell types may be involved in some way or another, and there may be many interactions between the different cells and the mediators they release (Figs 1 and 2). The roles of some of these cells are highlighted below.

Mast cells and macrophages

For a long time, mast cells have been assumed to play a central role in the pathogenesis of inflammatory airway diseases such as asthma [2]. They are present in large numbers in the epithelium of asthmatic patients, even those with mild asthma [3]. Furthermore, significant increases in the numbers of mast cells have been found in bronchoalveolar lavage fluid of asthmatics compared with normal control patients [4]. When degranulated, they are often surrounded by an area of damage, supporting the idea that these cells are active and are involved at least in the initial stages of the disease. Mast cells are often found in the epithelium with one surface adjacent to the airway lumen, and are in an ideal position to come into contact with inhaled antigens or a cold air challenge, and to release their mediators via an immunoglobulin (Ig)E-dependent mechanism both into the lumen of the airway and into the airway mucosa. The mediators released from mast cells include histamine, prostaglandin (PG)D_2 and a number of sulphidopeptide leukotrienes. Many of these agents are potent bronchoconstrictors and may be responsible for the rapid increase in airways resistance with allergic and other challenges to asthmatic airways. More importantly, these mediators may contribute by several mechanisms to the later inflammation and mucosal damage associated with the disease. Histamine is a vasodilator of the tracheobronchial circulation

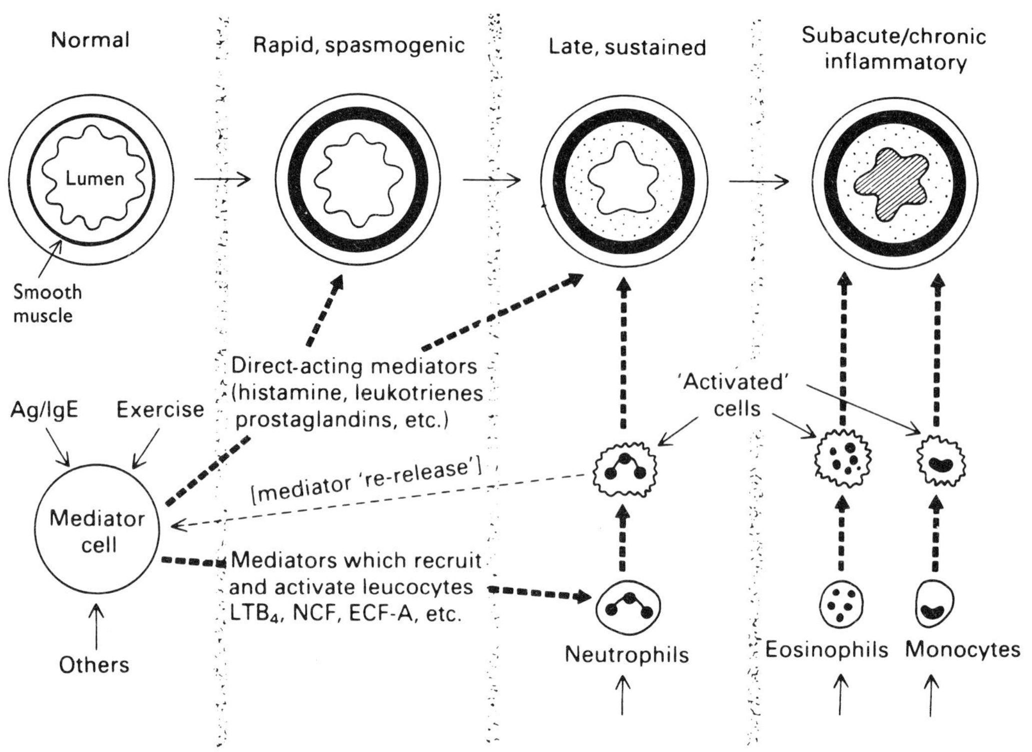

Fig. 1. Mediators, inflammatory cells and changes in the airway lumen during the progression of asthma

A cross-section of a bronchus is shown, with lumen surrounded by epithelium and a deeper layer of smooth muscle. Abbreviations used: Ag/IgE, antigen/immunoglobulin reaction; LTB_4, leukotriene B_4; NCF, neutrophil chemotactic factor; ECF-A, eosinophil chemotactic factor.

[5], and histamine and leukotrienes C_4, D_4 and E_4 all increase microvascular leakage and extravasation of proteins from airway blood vessels (see below for role of the vasculature); this latter effect is markedly potentiated by PGD_2 [6]. These mediators may also act directly on epithelial layers to increase their permeability. In addition, PGD_2 can further enhance the release of histamine from mast cells and basophils thereby increasing the response. PGD_2 is also weakly chemotactic for neutrophils and eosinophils. Following mast cell degranulation, however, other more potent chemotactic agents are released. These include eosinophil chemotactic factors of anaphylaxis and intermediate-molecular-weight eosinophil chemotactic factors. These agents together with PGD_2 will attract other inflammatory cells, particularly eosinophils, into the airway mucosa and perpetuate the inflammatory response and initiate mucosal and epithelial damage (see below).

Apart from mast cells, macrophages have been implicated in the immediate asthmatic response and the development of inflammation [7]. They are abundant throughout the respiratory tract, and recent evidence suggests that they may be activated by IgE-dependent mechanisms, indicating a role for them in allergic asthma [8]. When activated they release a number of mediators, including thromboxane, and a number of prostaglandins. However, perhaps the most important response of these cells is to release the mediator platelet-activating factor (PAF). The release of PAF from macrophages is greater in asthmatics than in normal controls and it seems to play a central role in the development of inflammation and mucosal damage in asthma. PAF is one of the most potent bronchoconstrictors known. More importantly, it is a potent vasodilator of the tracheobronchial circulation and it induces microvascular leakage from airway blood vessels. There is also some evidence that PAF can directly disrupt the bronchial epithelium and damage epithelial cells. Most importantly, PAF activates a wide range of inflammatory cells to release mediators which are extremely potent at causing inflammation and mucosal damage [9]. Of particular importance is its chemoattractant effect on the eosinophil and its ability to induce the release of toxic proteins from these cells (see below).

Eosinophils

For more than 80 years it has been known that bronchial asthma is often associated with eosinophilia of the blood and lung, and it seems that the connection between airway inflammation and mucosal damage and the eosinophil granulocyte is fundamental to the disease [10]. In groups of asthmatic patients the severity of the inflammatory disease correlates well with the blood eosinophil count, and in individuals the blood eosinophil count varies in relation to the severity of the disease. Thus, the eosinophil seems to be a marker of the extent of inflammation in asthmatics. In patients that respond to allergen challenge only with an early asthmatic reaction (1–2 h) there is no increase in blood or bronchoalveolar lavage eosinophils; however, in those which show a late-phase reaction, there is a corresponding increase in the number of eosinophils in lavage fluid after 6 h and in the blood after 24 h. Histologically there is evidence that the influx of eosinophils into the airway mucosa beneath the epithelium seems to be a characteristic

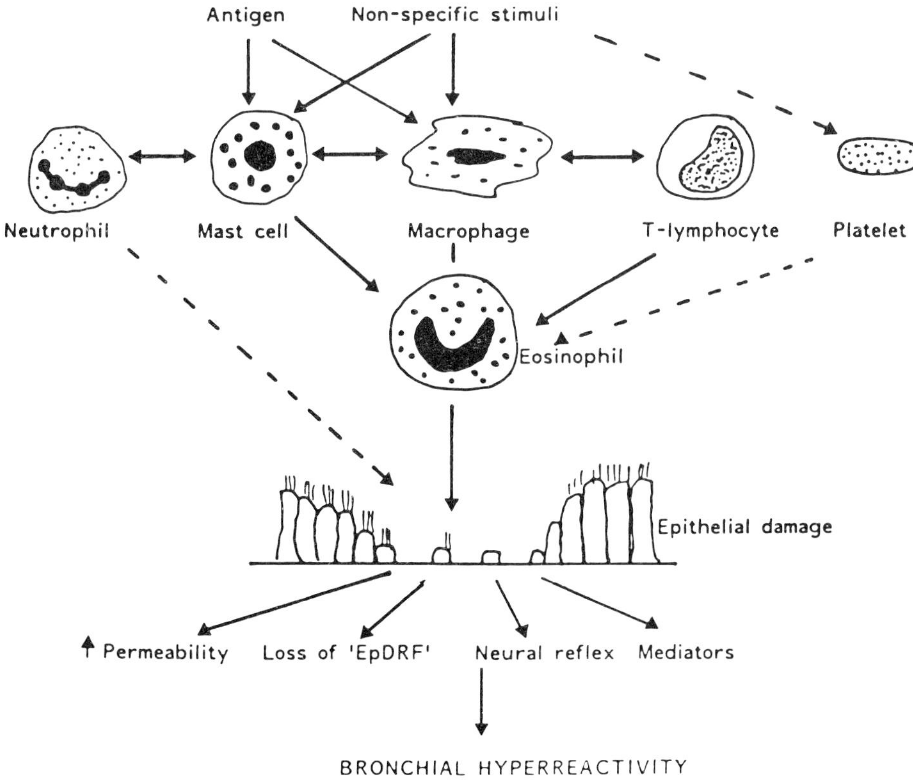

Fig. 2. Complex interactions between inflammatory cells may lead to structural changes such as epithelial shedding in the airways

This shedding, by several mechanisms, leads to a perpetuation of the inflammation. Solid arrows show established actions, interrupted arrows show possible actions, and double arrows show interactions. Figure reproduced by kind permission from [14].

feature of the disease, and the number of eosinophils in the bronchia mucosa is related to the deterioration of the asthma symptoms [11, 12]. Eosinophils may thus contribute to the pathophysiological process responsible for the change of stable asthma into an asthma attack.

When in the bronchial mucosa, the eosinophils can be stimulated (e.g. by PAF) to release a number of mediators including leukotriene C_4, PAF and oxygen free-radicals [9, 13]. These mediators are all pro-inflammatory, producing vasodilation, vascular leakage and submucosal gland secretion [14, 15]. In addition PAF is a potent chemoattractant for eosinophils (see above), and PAF and oxygen free-radicals can cause disruption and damage of the epithelium and may thicken the basement membrane (see below).

More importantly, eosinophils release a number of cytotoxic proteins from their granules [16]. There are at least four of these proteins — eosinophil cationic protein (ECP), eosinophil major basic protein (MBP), eosinophil-derived neurotoxin and eosinophil peroxidase. ECP seems to be by far the most potent tissue-damaging protein produced by the eosinophils. A single injection into the guinea-pig trachea of 0.2–0.5 μg ECP produces damage to the surface epithelium. This damage varies from detachment of the superficial part of the epithelium, leaving behind intact basal cells, to a total removal of the epithelium in other places, especially those near the site of injection. Immunoreactivity to ECP has been correlated to cellular injury in post-mortem lungs from asthmatics. Where ECP activity is restricted to inside eosinophils there is no cellular injury; however, where eosinophils have degranulated, the extracellular ECP is always seen in or near damaged areas. Preliminary results suggest a similar correlation in living severe asthmatics. Extracellular ECP immunoreactivity is often seen throughout the bronchial wall as well as on the mucosal surface, and is associated with areas of mucosal destruction and ulceration. MBP can also induce epithelial damage and desquamation similar to the pathological changes in asthma (see below), and immunofluorescence for MBP is often deposited at sites of damage to bronchial epithelium, in mucus plugs, and in amorphous deposits beneath the epithelium in specimens of patients dying from asthma.

► The infiltration of inflammatory cells into the airway mucosa and lumen, and the subsequent release of various mediators, are the key events in the development of inflammation and mucosal damage in asthma.
► Mast cells and macrophages are implicated in the first stage of asthma; these cells release a number of bronchoconstrictors, the most potent being PAF.
► Eosinophils appear to be involved in the transition of stable asthma into an asthma attack, their concentration varying in relation to the severity of the disease.
► Eosinophils are stimulated by e.g. PAF to release pro-inflammatory mediators and a number of cytotoxic proteins, the most potent being ECP.

Changes in epithelial and basement membrane structure

The epithelium of the mammalian bronchial tree is of the ciliated pseudostratified columnar type in the trachea and main bronchi and turns into a simple cuboidal type deep inside the lung [17]. The types of cell found in the bronchial epithelium differ according to species. In the human, four main cells — ciliated cells, basal cells, secretory (mucous or goblet) cells and Kulchitsky (neuroendocrine, amine-containing, APUD or K) cells — all rest on a basement membrane. Ciliated, secretory and K cells all reach the lumen of the airway and there are three to five ciliated cells for every mucous cell. The epithelium also contains a few lymphocytes and nerve profiles (see below) near the lumen and basement membrane.

The epithelium, being adjacent to the airway lumen, is a prime target organ for exogenous irritants such as allergens, bacteria and viruses, and for mediators released by inflammatory cells into the lumen (Fig. 2, see above). One of the characteristic features of inflammatory airway diseases such as asthma is disruption and shedding of the airway epithelium; indeed, at the end stage of asthma in specimens from patients dying in status asthmaticus, it is extremely difficult to find normal areas of bronchial epithelium [18].

Considerable problems have been encountered in studying the structural changes in the epithelium in living asthmatic patients, mainly because of the difficulty in obtaining representative specimens of the human airways. One attempt to overcome this problem was the examination of the sputum of asthmatic patients, the presence of stripped respiratory epithelial cells being one of the first pathological abnormalities detected in this disease [19]. Later, the term 'Creola body' was introduced to describe large sheets of exfoliated epithelium that condense to form spherical or elongated masses in the overlying mucous layer. More recent studies have concentrated on measuring immunoglobulin levels and eosinophil-derived products in sputum, both of these being enhanced in asthmatics [20]. The technique of bronchoalveolar lavage has also been used to assess the cell population present in the lumen of the airways of both healthy subjects and asthmatics. This consists of washing saline into part of the lung through a bronchoscope, and then withdrawing it for analysis. Epithelial cell numbers, as well as the numbers of other inflammatory cells (see above), are increased in the asthmatics.

More recently, the development of fibre-optic (flexible) bronchoscopy has meant that biopsy material can be taken from the lungs and airways of living asthmatics; this, together with great improvements in light and electron microscopic techniques, has enabled a more detailed analysis of the changes in airway mucosal structure in living asthmatics [21]. One of the most prominent features in these patients is a marked airway oedema with separation of the epithelial cells, leaving behind in many areas only a layer of basal or reserve cells. The epithelium often has a fragile appearance, caused either by shedding of the columnar epithelial cells or by intracellular signs of destruction such as vacuolization of the endoplasmic reticulum. Where epithelial shedding is present there is also an accumulation of homogeneous mass, probably oedema fluid, in the widened intracellular spaces at the base of the epithelium. This homogeneous mass pushes the uppermost columnar epithelial cells away, and this process can be seen most often close to regions of extensive epithelial destruction, such as in areas where only the basal cells are present or where the basement membrane is totally denuded. Despite this destructive separation process, the columnar epithelial cells may have a quite normal appearance, still being attached together at the luminal side by the tight junctions. Epithelial shedding is a commonly described feature of asthma and is one of the first features described in airway pathological changes of asthma. Other cellular changes not so regularly reported are goblet cell hyperplasia and epithelial cell metaplasia. These changes may be related to airway epithelial degeneration and regeneration processes.

The majority of studies have shown the basement membrane to be thickened in asthmatic patients, particularly where there is evidence of epithelial cell shedding [22]. Fibronectin refers to a group of structurally and immunologically related high-molecular-weight glycoproteins present in plasma and extracellular matrix. It is thought to be important in cell–cell and cell–matrix interactions and, together with fibrin, is a temporary component of the extracellular matrix in the basement membrane during healing of epithelial damage. The location of fibronectin in the mucosa of non-smoking asthmatics was studied using immunofluorescence techniques. The basement membrane of these patients was thickened and fibronectin was revealed as a bright reaction in the basement membrane underneath areas of epithelial shedding or adjacent to the edge of ulcerated epithelium. In control subjects, the fibronectin reaction was negative.

Consequences of epithelial damage

Damage to or shedding of the respiratory epithelium is likely to have important consequences for both the pathophysiology and treatment of asthma (Fig. 2). Most importantly, the loss of epithelium is going to lead, by a variety of mechanisms, to the perpetuation and proliferation of the inflammation and mucosal damage associated with the disease. These mechanisms include:

— (i) increased permeability of the airway to inhaled irritants, bacteria and viruses, and mediators released from inflammatory cells into the lumen

— (ii) exposure of sensory nerves, neuroepithelial bodies and neuroendocrine-like cells in the epithelium

— (iii) loss of epithelial protective functions including loss of inhibitory factors released from epithelial cells
— (iv) increased release of inflammatory mediators from damaged epithelium.

Changes in epithelial permeability

An increase in the size of the paracellular junctions between epithelial cells or loss of the epithelial cells altogether is likely to lead to increased permeability of the airway mucosa to inflammatory mediators released into the airway lumen, allergens and bacteria, and thus to a proliferation of the inflammation [23]. This increase in permeability may be brought about by the inflammatory mediators themselves, particularly toxic proteins released from eosinophils (see above), or by luminal stimuli such as hypertonicity of the airway lining fluid which disrupts epithelial tight junctions [24]. Evidence for increased permeability in asthmatics is lacking; however, animal studies have shown that PAF reduces transepithelial tracheal potential difference, indicating epithelial disruption, while increasing permeability to agents of small molecular weight placed in the airway lumen.

Exposure of sensory nerves and release of sensory peptides

Nerves in the epithelium are usually near to the basal lamina. On the basis of ultrastructural and other criteria these nerves contain many mitochondria and are therefore thought to be afferent or sensory [25]. At places where there is epithelial damage and shedding, these nerves will become exposed and can be stimulated by a number of luminal irritants and mediators. Furthermore, the loss of epithelium means there is a direct passage between the lumen and the submucosal tissues where there are further nerve endings. If these afferent nerves are stimulated antidromically by luminal agents, this leads to the release of sensory peptides [substance P (SP), neurokinin A (NKA), neurokinin B (NKB), calcitonin gene-related peptide (CGRP)] by a local axon reflex into the mucosa. These peptides are potent bronchoconstrictors (particularly NKA) and vasodilators (particularly CGRP), and they induce microvascular leakage, plasma exudation and submucosal gland secretion (particularly SP) [14, 15]. They can also activate inflammatory cells, including epithelial cells, to cause a further release of mediators. This process is known as neurogenic inflammation, although the pathways for the local axon reflexes have not been established histologically.

Neuroepithelial bodies and neuroendocrine cells in the epithelium

Apart from nerves, there are two other types of cell in the epithelium which may be activated during airway inflammation. These cells are individual granule-containing cells (also referred to as Feyrter cells, Kulchitsky cells, argyrophil, fluorescent and granulated cells, neuroendocrine-like cells and APUD cells), as well as groups of similar cells defined as neuroepithelial bodies [26]. Both the single cells and the neuroepithelial bodies have been found in a number of species including humans, and cells of both types have a triangular shape which rests on the basement membrane. The larger basal part of the cell often contains many dense-cored vesicles. Afferent nerve profiles have been observed close to single granule-containing cells. Either a neural stimulation or a stimulus from the airway lumen (particularly when there is epithelial damage) may cause these cells to release amines or neuropeptides into the mucosa thereby perpetuating the inflammation.

Loss of epithelial protection

Recently, several studies have shown that damage to or removal of the epithelium enhances the effects of spasmogens on the airway smooth muscle and secretagogues on the submucosal glands. In addition, the effectiveness of some bronchodilator drugs is reduced. The enhanced bronchoconstriction could be explained by increased access of a luminal spasmogen or secretagogue to the smooth muscle or glands because of the missing epithelium, although such an explanation could not account for the reduced effect of the bronchodilators. A further possibility is that epithelial cells are important for the uptake and/or degradation of released mediators; thus, if the cells are removed this might prolong the action of the mediators. Indeed, the enkephalinase enzymes primarily responsible for the breakdown of sensory peptides are found in a high concentration in the epithelium. If the epithelium is stripped, these enzymes will be removed and the effectiveness of the sensory peptides in perpetuating the inflammatory response will be increased. However, this explanation cannot account for an increased responsiveness to acetylcholine since the presence of acetylcholinesterase inhibitors does not diminish this effect. A further possibility is that the epithelial cells release one or more inhibitory factors which may act to reduce smooth muscle tone, in a manner similar to endothelial-derived relaxing factor (EDRF) released from vascular endothelial cells. The identity of this putative epithelial-derived relaxing factor (EpDRF) has not yet been established [27], but it is unlikely to be the same as EDRF since agents which inhibit this factor have no effect on EpDRF. Similar or different inhibitory factors may be released from epithelial cells which modulate gland secretion and blood flow, although evidence for a functional role for these mediators is lacking at present.

Release of mediators from damaged epithelium

There are a number of mediators released from epithelial cells themselves which could perpetuate the inflammation and mucosal damage associated with asthma. These include prostaglandins, leukotrienes, 15-hydroxyeicosatetraenoic acid (15-HETE; particularly from human cells) and the endothelins [28]. Damage to epithelial cells may lead to a transient increase in release of these mediators which may result in secondary cell recruitment and increase the inflammatory reaction.

- ► Shedding of the airway epithelial cells is a common feature of asthma, and in damaged areas the basement membrane is thickened.
- ► At sites of epithelial damage, the airway mucosa is more permeable to inflammatory mediators, allergens and bacteria, and neurogenic inflammation may also occur.
- ► A further consequence of loss of epithelial protection is that spasmogens and secretagogues will have increased access to the airway smooth muscle and submucosal glands, respectively, thus enhancing their effects.

Role of the airways circulation in mucosal damage

The tracheobronchial circulation is essential for maintaining the normal functions of the tissues of the airways mucosa [29]. While airways blood flow comprises only a few percent of cardiac output, weight-for-weight mucosal blood flow is extremely high at around 100 ml min^{-1} 100 g^{-1}. Arteries and arterioles supply a dense subepithelial capillary network which extends along the length of the airways in the mucosa, the capillaries draining via a deeper venous plexus [30]. Submucosal glands have an extensive capillary supply, but airways smooth muscle has a sparse vasculature. The endothelium unlike that in the nose is non-fenestrated. A second capillary network is present outside the smooth muscle of the bronchi in the peribronchial space and is connected to the first by vessels running through the muscle layer.

It is becoming clear that the circulation plays a significant role in the development of airway inflammation and mucosal damage (Fig. 3). It is the source of many inflammatory cell types and mediators and the means by which they will reach sites of tissue damage or inflammation. In sheep and pigs that have spontaneous development of allergy to foreign proteins, inhalation of allergen produces a rapid increase in tracheobronchial blood flow in parallel with the changes in airways function [31]. In sheep, a second increase in blood flow has been demonstrated that occurs about 5 h after challenge and precedes the 'late' changes in airways function. Increased microvascular leakage, tissue oedema and plasma exudation into the airways lumen are also associated with allergen challenge.

Microvascular leakage and plasma exudation

Normally the airways vascular bed is almost impermeable to plasma protein and macromolecules. Fluid flux between the vasculature and the interstitium is determined by the hydrostatic pressure gradient across the capillary wall driving fluid out, and by the oncotic pressure of plasma opposing this. There is a small net flow of fluid into the interstitium that is removed from the tissue by the lymphatic system.

Inflammatory agents can increase microvascular permeability so that plasma proteins enter the interstitium. The leakage of protein will substantially reduce the oncotic pressure gradient and enhance fluid flux into the interstitium. As fluid flux into the tissue exceeds fluid removal oedema will develop. Histamine, bradykinin, PAF, leukotrienes and SP are all agents that produce microvascular leakage.

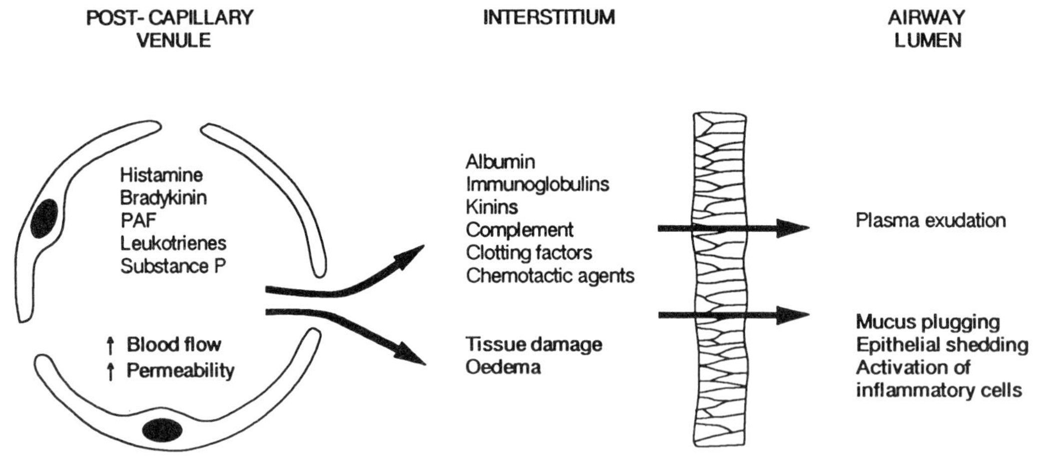

Fig. 3. The role of the vasculature in the development of airway inflammation and structural damage

In inflammation the site of the leakage is not the capillary bed but the post-capillary venules. Inflammatory agents open gaps in the endothelial lining of the venules which allow the passage of large molecules into the interstitium. It appears that the gaps are opened by the actions of the endothelial cells which contain contractile elements. Ultrastructural studies of airway vessels from asthmatics show evidence of such endothelial gap formation. It is worth noting that white cell infiltration of inflamed tissue can occur independently of microvascular leakage; these cells can pass through the endothelium into the interstitium through 'leak-free' channels.

Increasing blood flow alone appears to have little effect on microvascular leakage. Agents such as CGRP and methacholine can cause vasodilation without affecting endothelial permeability and do not produce microvascular leakage. However, it has been shown clearly in skin that such agents, presumably by increasing microvascular hydrostatic pressure, can substantially magnify leakage produced by other agents. Conversely, vasoconstrictors can reduce the degree of microvascular leakage produced by these agents. Most inflammatory agents do themselves increase mucosal blood flow [31].

Following microvascular leakage, plasma proteins and macromolecules can be detected in the fluid of the airways lumen: this phenomenon is described as plasma exudation [32]. It appears that plasma is exuded into the lumen through the paracellular spaces of the epithelium. While this can occur without disruption of the epithelium it is likely that the fluid flux and increased interstitial hydrostatic pressure will contribute to epithelial shedding.

Extravasated plasma will contain many factors not normally present in the tissue, including albumin, immunoglobulins, kinins, complement, clotting factors and chemotactic agents. These may lead to local tissue damage and activation of inflammatory cells. Tissue oedema itself is hard to quantify and most airways studies have measured changes in permeability and not changes in the volume of fluid. However, oedema is clearly evident in inflamed airways, and the tissue swelling it produces can lead directly to airways obstruction. Oedema in the peribronchial spaces may affect the elastic recoil forces that keep the small airways open and alter lung compliance. The condition is only resolved slowly by lymphatic drainage and it is possible that plasma exudation into the airways lumen is a route that will allow more rapid clearance of interstitial fluid.

Plasma exuded into the lumen will not be harmless, however. It will increase mucus viscosity, enhance the formation of mucus plugs and impair mucociliary transport. Plasma proteins may also be important for activating inflammatory cells in the lumen. It is possible that albumin has a protective anti-oxidant action. However, plasma exudation is not the only source of albumin, as it can be actively secreted into the lumen, probably by the epithelium.

Increased microvascular permeability and plasma exudation can be reduced by the actions of anti-asthma drugs; this may be a major aspect of the success of these drugs in treating the disease [33]. Glucocorticoids and sodium cromoglycate both reduce plasma exudation. PAF antagonists may also be effective in reducing antigen-induced plasma leakage. It is interesting that β-agonists, used therapeutically as smooth muscle relaxants, also appear to possess anti-inflammatory activity; they may act directly on the post-capillary venular endothelium to reduce vascular permeability.

Other roles of the circulation

Blood flow may also alter the distribution and removal of substances from the airways wall, thus disrupting their actions [34]. Both harmful substances, such as allergen, and therapeutic agents, such as smooth muscle relaxants, may be inhaled and absorbed into the airways. Once they have passed through the epithelium and interstitium they will enter the capillary bed. Similarly, endogenous mediators released from inflammatory cells will diffuse into the circulation. Once in the vasculature these agents may be redistributed into the other airway tissues or removed completely from the airways. Changes in blood flow may modulate both uptake and distribution and therefore the actions of these agents on the airways mucosa. The effect of blood flow in modulating mucosal damage has not itself been studied. However, decreasing bronchial blood flow increases the duration of both histamine and methacholine-induced bronchoconstriction in anaesthetized animals. Decreasing tracheal mucosal blood flow with vasopressin prolongs smooth muscle constriction produced with antigen, while increasing blood flow can abolish the effects. Similar effects of blood flow on actions within the mucosa might be expected. However, in judging the benefit of such actions, it must be remembered that increasing blood flow may also enhance microvascular leakage.

Drugs used to treat airways disease may themselves alter airway blood flow and therefore, in effect, modify their own actions. Salbutamol, a smooth muscle relaxant, dilates the tracheobronchial circulation; adrenaline, while not generally used to treat asthma, is an example of an agent that relaxes airways smooth muscle and constricts the circulation.

The endothelium itself should not be forgotten for it is the source of many agents that may influence mucosal damage. PAF, endothelin, prostaglandins and chemotactic factors are all produced by endothelial cells and have inflammatory or pro-inflammatory actions.

Repair of inflammatory changes in the bronchial mucosa

The mechanism underlying the turnover and repair of the respiratory epithelium is not well understood. Ciliated cells are easily damaged and loss of these cells is an early response to many forms of injury [35]. These cells are end-stage cells and contain no DNA and do not divide; they are not replaced until the adverse situation or damaging stimulus is removed. When the epithelium is damaged it is the mucous cells and the basal cells which proliferate. It is widely assumed that it is the basal cells which are responsible for regeneration of the epithelium. However, recently it has been suggested that mucous cells may play the dominant role in proliferation [36]. Resulting from a marked increase in the mitotic rate of these cells, pathological lesions including goblet cell hyperplasia, stratification and non-cornifying and cornifying epidermoid (squamous) metaplasias may be produced. Although morphologically distinct, these lesions are brought about by the wide and varied spectrum of the phenotypic expression of mucous cells. Depending on the extent of the injury, one or more of these lesions may be present and one lesion may turn into another. Both basal and mucous cells synthesize DNA, yet the extent to which each cell type is involved in the regeneration process is not clear. Stimulated ciliogenesis may be one step in the regeneration of the epithelium. The number of cells with fibrogranular areas, which are precursors in cilia formation, increases in asthmatic patients treated with steroids. Fibronectin may play an important role in the regeneration and healing process. It has been detected in asthmatic subjects at the site of bronchial epithelial regeneration, which is comparable to the location of fibronectin in other damaged human epithelia (e.g. in the gut). This provides evidence of a wound-healing role for fibronectin in the airways.

> ▶ Inflammatory agents can increase microvascular permeability so that plasma proteins enter the interstitium; this is known as 'microvascular leakage' and results in oedema.
> ▶ Plasma exudation into the airways lumen may occur following microvascular leakage.
> ▶ Epithelium regeneration is brought about primarily by proliferation of basal cells and mucous cells.
> ▶ Fibronectin, located in the basement membrane of asthmatics, is thought to play a major wound-healing role

Conclusions

Despite a huge amount of research into the mechanisms underlying asthma many uncertainties remain. The development of inflammation and structural mucosal damage in asthmatics is obviously an extremely complex process with many interactions between mucosal tissues, inflammatory cells and inflammatory mediators. The inflammation is characterized by infiltration of a number of different inflammatory cells and the excessive release of numerous mediators. These mediators act on the target tissues to cause hypersecretion of mucus, vasodilation, increased vascular permeability and structural changes in the mucosa. There is still considerable debate as to which cells and which mediators are the most important for the development and proliferation of the inflammation. It seems likely that eosinophils, through the release of pro-inflammatory mediators such as PAF and oxygen free-radicals, and toxic proteins such as ECP and MBP, are responsible for much of the cellular injury related to asthma. This damage is mainly to the surface epithelium but may even be seen in deeper structures. Of the mediators, PAF appears to be very important, and the animal models to which exogenous PAF has been administered mimic many of the features of asthma. The mucosal structural damage, particularly to the epithelium, leads by a variety of mechanisms to the perpetuation and proliferation of the inflammation associated with asthma.

Thus, although we understand many of the inflammatory processes occurring in asthma, and we can suggest ways in which the mucosal damage could occur, there are many questions still to be answered:

— the interactions between inflammatory cells are not well understood
— it is not clear if the epithelial damage precedes or is a consequence of cellular infiltration
— the exact role of the numerous mediators released during the inflammation is far from established.

Finally, perhaps the most important problem is that the animal models which we use for trying to solve these questions may bear an uncertain resemblance to human asthma.

References

1. Kay, A. B. (1986) Mediators and inflammatory cells in asthma. In Asthma: Clinical Pharmacology and Therapeutic Progress (Kay, A. B., ed.), pp. 1–10, Blackwell Scientific Publications, Oxford
2. Holgate, S. T. and Kay, A. B. (1985) Mast cells, mediators and asthma. Clin. Allergy **15**, 221–234
3. Salvato, G. (1968) Asthma and mast cells of bronchial connective tissue. Experentia **18**, 330–331
4. Wardlaw, A. J., Dunnette, S., Gleich, G. J., Collins, J. V. and Kay, A. B. (1988) Eosinophils and mast cells in bronchoalveolar lavage in subjects with mild asthma. Am. Rev. Resp. Dis. **137**, 62–69
5. Webber, S. E., Salonen, R. O. and Widdicombe, J. G. (1988) H1 and H2-receptor characterisation in the tracheal circulation of sheep. Br. J. Pharmacol. **95**, 551–561
6. Hua, X. Y., Dahlen, S. E., Lundberg, J. M., Hammerstorm, S. and Hedquist, P. (1985) Leukotrienes C4 and E4 cause widespread and extensive plasma extravasation in the guinea-pig. Naunyn-Schmeideberg's Arch. Int. Pharmacodyn. **330**, 136–141
7. Macdermott, J. and Fuller, R. W. (1988) Macrophages. In Asthma: Basic Mechanisms and Clinical Management (Barnes, P. J., Rodger, I. W. and Thomson, N. C., eds.), pp. 97–114, Academic Press, London
8. Joseph, M., Tonnel, A. B., Tarpier, G. and Capron, A. (1983) Involvement of immunoglobulin E in the secretory process of alveolar macrophages from asthmatic patients. J. Clin. Invest. **71**, 221–230
9. Lee, T. C., Lenihan, D. J., Malone, B., Roddy, L. L. and Wasserman, S. I. (1984) Increased biosynthesis of platelet-activating factor in activated human eosinophils. J. Biol. Chem. **259**, 5526–5530
10. Burrows, B., Hasan, F. M., Barbree, R. M., Halonen, M. and Lecrowitz, M. D. (1980) Epidemiological observations on eosinophilia and its relation to respiratory diseases. Am. Rev. Resp. Dis. **122**, 709–712
11. Dunnill, M. S. (1960) The pathology of asthma with special reference to changes in the bronchial mucosa. J. Clin. Pathol. **13**, 27–33

12. Durham, S. R. and Kay, A. B. (1985) Eosinophils, bronchial reactivity and late asthmatic reactions. Clin. Allergy 40, 411–418
13. Shaw, R. J., Cromwell, O. and Kay, A. B. (1984) Preferential generation of leukotriene C4 by human eosinophils. Clin. Exp. Immunol. 70, 716–722
14. Barnes, P. J., Rodger, I. W. and Thomson, N. C. (1988) Pathogenesis of asthma. In Asthma: Basic Mechanisms and Clinical Management (Barnes, P. J., Rodger, I. W. and Thomson, N. C., eds.), pp. 415–444, Academic Press, London
15. Barnes, P. J., Chung, K. F. and Page, C. P. (1988) Inflammatory mediators and asthma. Pharmacol. Rev. 40, 49–84
16. Dahl, R., Venge, P. and Fredens, K. (1988) Eosinophils. In Asthma: Basic Mechanisms and Clinical Management (Barnes, P. J., Rodger, I. W. and Thomson, N. C., eds.), pp. 115–130, Academic Press, London
17. Rhodin, J. A. G. (1974) Respiratory System. In Histology, pp. 607–645, Oxford University Press, New York/London/Toronto
18. Dunnill, M. S. (1982) Pulmonary Pathology, Churchill Livingstone, New York
19. Curshmann, H. (1885) Einege Bernerkungen uber die im Bronchialsecret vorkommenden Spiralen. Dtsch. Arch. Klin. Med. 36, 578–585
20. Dor, P. J., Ackerman, S. J. and Gleich, G. J. (1984) Charcot-Leyden crystal protein and eosinophil granule major basic protein in sputum of patients with respiratory disease. Am. Rev. Resp. Dis. 130, 1072–1077
21. Laitinen, L. A., Heino, M., Laitinen, A., Kava, T. and Haahtela, T. (1985) Damage of the airway epithelium and bronchial reactivity in patients with asthma. Am. Rev. Resp. Dis. 131, 599–606
22. Beasley, R., Roche, W. R., Roberts, J. A. and Holgate, S. T. (1989) Cellular events in the bronchi in mild asthma and after bronchial provocation. Am. Rev. Resp. Dis. 139, 806–817
23. Hogg, J. C. (1981) Bronchial mucosal permeability and its relationship to airway hyperreactivity. J. Allergy Clin. Immunol. 67, 421–426
24. Hogg, J. C. and Eggleston, P. A. (1984) Is asthma an epithelial disease? Am. Rev. Resp. Dis. 129, 207–208
25. Das, R. M., Jeffery, P. K. and Widdicombe, J. G. (1979) Experimental degeneration of intra-epithelial nerve fibres in cat airways. J. Anat. 128, 259–267
26. Lauweryns, J. M. and Peuskens, J. C. (1972) Neuro-epithelial bodies (neuro-receptor or secretory organs?) in human infant bronchial and bronchiolar epithelium. Am. Rev. Resp. Dis. 172, 471–482
27. Flavahan, N. A. and Vanhoutte, P. M. (1985) The respiratory epithelium releases a smooth muscle relaxing factor. Chest 87, 1895–1905
28. Hunter, J. A., Finkbeiner, W. E., Nadel, J. A., Goetzl, E. J. and Holtzman, M. J. (1985) Predominant generation of 15-lipoxygenase metabolites of arachidonic acid by epithelial cells from human trachea. Proc. Natl. Acad. Sci. U.S.A. 82, 4633–4637
29. Wanner, A. (1989) Circulation of the airway mucosa. J. Appl. Physiol. 67, 917–925
30. Laitinen, A. and Laitinen, L. A. (1990) Vascular beds in the airways of normal man and asthmatics. Eur. Resp. J. 3 (Suppl. 12), 658–662
31. Webber, S. E., Salonen, R. O., Corfield, D. R. and Widdicombe, J. G. (1990) Effects of non-neural mediators and allergen on tracheobronchial blood flow. Eur. Resp. J. 3 (Suppl. 12), 638–644
32. Persson, C. G. A. (1991) Tracheobronchial microcirculation in asthma. In Asthma, its Pathology and Treatment (Kaliner, M. A., Barnes, P. J. and Persson, C. G. A., eds.), pp. 209–229, Marcel Dekker, New York
33. Barnes, P. J., Boschetto, P., Rogers, D. F., Belvisi, M., Roberts, N., Chung, K. F. and Evans, T. (1990) Effects of treatment on airway microvascular leak. Eur. Resp. J. 3 (Suppl. 12), 663–671
34. Wagner, E. M. and Mitzner, W. A. (1990) Bronchial circulatory reversal of methacholine-induced airway obstruction. J. Appl. Physiol. 69, 1220–1224
35. McDowell, E. M., Becci, P. J., Schurch, W. and Trump, F. F. (1979) The respiratory epithelium. VII. Epidermoid metaplasia of hamster tracheal epithelium during regeneration following mechanical injury. J. Natl. Cancer Inst. 62, 995–1008
36. McDowell, E. M. and Beals, T. F. (1987) Biopsy Pathology of the Bronchi, W. B. Saunders, Philadelphia

9

The pathophysiology of gastric and duodenal ulcer

John L. Wallace, Paula M. Vaananen and Cory M. Hogaboam
Gastrointestinal Research Group, University of Calgary, Calgary, Alberta T2N 4N1, Canada

Introduction

Ulceration of the gastric and duodenal mucosa represents an important clinical concern, and contributes significantly to the financial burden of health care systems. Important advances in the treatment of these diseases have been made over the past two decades, and these have resulted in a decrease in the incidence of peptic ulcer disease [1]. Despite these advances, however, the pathogenesis of ulceration remains obscure.

In order to understand why the gastric or duodenal mucosae become injured under certain circumstances, it is first necessary to ascertain how and why the mucosa is resistant to damage under normal circumstances. The upper gastro-intestinal tract is almost continually exposed to potentially noxious agents, including endogenous substances (hydrochloric acid, pepsins, bile salts) and those substances which we ingest. Some of the substances we ingest may be capable of irritating the mucosa by virtue of high temperatures or high osmolarity, while other substances can damage mucosal cells because of their ability to disrupt membranes (e.g. ethanol) or inhibit cellular metabolism (e.g. aspirin). It appears that the mucosa of the upper gastro-intestinal tract can withstand such exposure because of an elaborate set of defensive systems. Ulceration of the mucosa, therefore, may occur because of a failure of one or more of the components of this defence system.

In this chapter we will review the various components of the mucosal defence system and identify the response of the mucosa when one or more of these components fails. The factors that can contribute to or cause ulceration will be discussed, with particular reference to their effects on mucosal defence. In addition, the drugs which have been shown to be effective in the treatment of ulcer disease and their proposed mechanisms of action will be considered.

The mucosal defence system

The various components of the mucosal defence system can be said to be organized in a hierarchical manner [2]. If one component is overcome by irritants present in the lumen, the next level of defence is called into play. Some of the components of mucosal defence are illustrated in Fig. 1. Paradoxically, the first component of mucosal defence is actually an endogenous 'aggressive' factor — acid. Acid appears to be very important as a bactericidal agent, reducing the entry into the intestine of microbes ingested with meals. The importance of this role of acid is underscored by reports in the literature that the incidence of diarrhoea is increased significantly in patients taking constant high doses of inhibitors of gastric acid secretion (histamine H_2 receptor antagonists). Interestingly, there is now strong evidence that some forms of peptic ulcer disease may be related to colonization of the stomach by the bacterium *Helicobacter pylori.* This bacterium is specially adapted so that it can survive in an environment in which the pH is extremely low (see below).

The mucus secreted onto the surface of the gastric and duodenal epithelium also serves as an important protective barrier against invasion of the mucosa by microbes. These organisms become trapped in mucus and are then carried through the gastro-intestinal tract and excreted. It is possible that mucus may play a role in protecting the gastroduodenal epithelium from damage induced by acid and pepsin, although this theory is somewhat con-

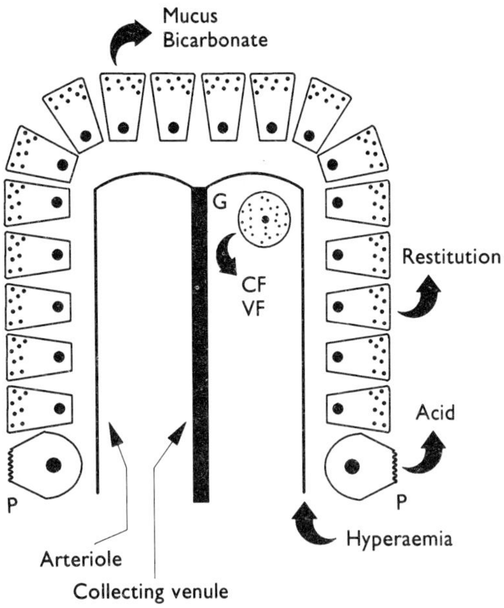

Fig. 1. Components of the mucosal defence system
Mucus and bicarbonate secreted by the surface epithelial cells may contribute to protecting those cells from damage induced by acid and pepsin. Acid secretion from parietal cells (P) plays an important microbicidal role. The surface epithelium may itself be specially adapted to resist damage by acid. When the epithelium is damaged, repair is rapid through migration of healthy cells from the gastric pits (restitution). This process is facilitated by release of mucus and efflux of plasma, creating a local microenvironment of relatively high pH. Mucosal blood flow increases substantially following superficial injury, mediated by release of vasoactive factors (VF) from sensory afferent nerves and from 'immune' cells in the lamina propria. These latter cells can also release chemotactic factors (CF) which will recruit granulocytes to the site of injury. The granulocytes (G) remove any foreign substances which crossed the breached epithelium, as well as playing an important role in clearing any necrotic tissue, so that repair can proceed.

troversial. It has been postulated that the mucus adherent to the epithelium traps bicarbonate secreted by those cells, creating a local microenvironment of relatively high pH [3].

It is possible that gastroduodenal epithelial cells are specially adapted to allow them to resist damage when exposed to high concentrations of acid. Consider the parietal cell, for instance. The concentration gradient of hydrogen ions across the membrane of this cell can exceed one million to one, yet the cell is seldom observed to be damaged by acid. The epithelial cells at the luminal surface of the mucosa are continuously extruded into the lumen and replaced by younger cells which migrate from the progenitor zone in the gastric pits, where cell division occurs. If injury to the surface epithelium occurs, a distinct type of cell replacement is initiated which is referred to as 'restitution' [4]. This process is independent of cell division and involves the movement of healthy cells from the gastric pits over the exposed basement membrane to re-establish an intact epithelium. Depending on the extent of injury, the process can be complete within 15 to 60 min, and therefore reduces the potential for entry into the mucosa of any microbes or foreign substances which might have deleterious effects.

While the role of mucus in protecting the mucosa from damage under normal conditions is controversial [5], there is clear evidence that the mucus released when the surface epithelium is damaged is very important in allowing the epithelium to be repaired before damage extends any further into the mucosa [6]. When the epithelium is damaged, a cap of mucus, fibrin and other plasma products forms over the damaged region (much like a scab on a cut). Even when the pH of the gastric lumen is below 1, the pH within this 'mucoid cap' can be maintained between 5 and 6. This microenvironment is very important because the basement membrane along which epithelial cells migrate is very susceptible to damage by acid. If this membrane is destroyed, rapid repair of superficial injury by restitution is impossible and much more severe injury to the mucosa can ensue.

Superficial injury to the gastric epithelium, or increased rates of diffusion of luminal acid into the mucosa (acid 'back-diffusion') elicit an elevation in mucosal blood flow. This reactive hyperaemia can be attributed to dilation of submucosal arterioles. More specifically, sensory afferent neurons with endings near the surface of the gastric mucosa can be activated by back-diffusing acid or toxins to release the vasodilator neurotransmitter calcitonin gene-related peptide (CGRP) in the region of the submucosal arterioles. The increase in blood flow which can be attributed to CGRP-induced vasodilation appears to be essential for adequate buffering of back-diffusing acid, and for the dilution and removal of toxins. This defensive response therefore limits the accumulation of potentially toxic substances within the mucosa, and, in doing so, limits the extent of injury to the most superficial layers of cells. There is considerable evidence that the reactive hyperaemia following injury is very important in permitting the damage to be repaired through restitution.

Prostaglandins are a group of fatty acids derived from membrane phospholipids which may also play an important role in mediating the reactive hyperaemic response to superficial damage [7]. Virtually every type of cell in the mucosa is capable of releasing prostaglandins in response to membrane perturbation. It is possible that the back-diffusion of acid or toxins stimulates local release of prostaglandins. These substances are potent vasodilators, so that the net result of their release is an increase in mucosal blood flow. Inhibitors of prostaglandin synthesis, such as aspirin or indomethacin, have been shown to attenuate the hyperaemic response to topical irritants, resulting in an exacerbation of the injury induced by the irritant [8]. It should be noted that prostaglandins may also affect other components of the mucosal defence system, including the secretion of mucus and bicarbonate and the acute inflammatory response (see below).

The acute inflammatory response is another component of the mucosal defence system which is brought into play following mucosal injury. Lying just beneath the epithelium, in the 'lamina propria', are a number of different types of cells capable of releasing mediators that can recruit circulating inflammatory cells into the interstitium. For example, mast cells, eosinophils and macrophages can release mediators that are chemotactic for granulocytes, increase mucosal blood flow and increase vascular permeability [9]. The infiltration of granulocytes into the lamina propria is aimed at preventing the entry into the systemic circulation of microbes, antigens or other foreign substances.

Table 1 lists some of the inflammatory mediators that have been shown, at least in experimental models, to influence mucosal integrity. As in any inflammatory reaction, the acute response to superficial gastro-duodenal injury can actually lead to an enhancement of damage to the mucosa. Many inflammatory mediators have vasoconstrictor actions and have been shown to increase the susceptibility of the mucosa to injury. Leukotriene C_4 and thomboxane A_2 are two such examples. It is not clear if the amounts of these mediators

Table 1 **Vasoactive mediators: effects on the gastric mucosa**

Mediator	Cellular sources	Effect on blood flow	Effect on vascular permeability	Effect on susceptibility to ulceration
Histamine	Mast cells	Increase	Increase	Increase/decrease
PAF	Mast/endothelial cells	Decrease	Increase	Increase
LTB_4	Neutrophils	No effect	No effect	No effect
LTC_4	Mast/eosinophils	Decrease	Increase	Increase
TXA_2	Platelets	Decrease	No effect	Increase
CGRP	Neurons	Increase	No effect	Decrease
ET	Endothelial cells	Decrease	Increase	Increase
NO	Endothelial cells	Increase	No effect	Decrease

Abbreviations used: CGRP, calcitonin gene-related peptide (released from sensory afferent neurons, and perhaps other types of nerves in the gastroduodenal mucosae); ET, endothelin; LT, leukotriene; NO, nitric oxide; PAF, platelet-activating factor; TX, thromboxane. The effects of some of these mediators have been reviewed in detail recently (see [9]).

released following mucosal injury are sufficient for them to produce a reduction in mucosal blood flow, and it is likely that their effects are counterbalanced by release of other mediators, such as histamine and prostaglandins, which are potent vasodilators. The granulocytes which infiltrate the mucosa in response to the release of chemotactic factors can also contribute to mucosal injury by virtue of the proteolytic enzymes and reactive oxygen metabolites they release upon activation.

One of the other important roles of the inflammatory response to injury relates to the repair of ulcers. For repair to occur, the mass of necrotic tissue at the base of the ulcer must be cleared by phagocytes (primarily neutrophils and macrophages). If the inflammatory response is inhibited, repair of the ulcer is delayed and there is an increased chance of infection and/or perforation. It has been suggested that the association of corticosteroid therapy and gastro-duodenal ulceration (an association which is controversial in itself) may be related to the ability of corticosteroids to inhibit many components of the acute inflammatory reaction.

In summary, the mucosal defence system is comprised of components (acid, mucus, surface epithelium) aimed at preventing damage and components aimed at limiting the extent of damage. When the epithelium is breached, several of the components are called into play (hyperaemia, restitution, acute inflammatory response) with the goals of rapidly restoring epithelial integrity and preventing entry of foreign substances into the systemic circulation.

- ▶ The various components of the mucosal defence system in the upper gastro-intestinal tract are organized in a hierarchical manner; failure of one or more of these components may result in ulceration.
- ▶ Acid acts as a bactericidal agent, while mucus provides a protective barrier against microbes.
- ▶ At sites of epithelial injury, 'restitution' (cell replacement by migration) occurs.
- ▶ Restitution is aided by the release of agents such as CGRP and prostaglandins which elicit a reactive hyperaemia response.
- ▶ The active inflammatory response involves the movement of circulatory inflammatory cells into the interstitium; these cells release mediators with various properties such as chemotaxis for granulocytes and increased vascular permeability.

Etiological factors

Helicobacter pylori

In recent years, a strong association between ulcer disease and *Helicobacter pylori* colonization of the stomach has become apparent [10] (see Table 2). For example, *H. pylori* can be detected in 67% and 90% of gastric and duodenal ulcer patients, respectively. In the extremely acidic environment of the stomach, it seems highly unlikely that any type of organism could survive, yet 50% of individuals over the age of 50 years test positive for *H. pylori*-like organisms. *H. pylori* (formerly called *Campylobacter pylori*) appears to avoid acid digestion by adhering to the antral and fundic mucosa of the stomach, beneath the layer of adherent mucus. This flagellated, gram-negative bacterium is non-invasive (it is incapable of entering the epithelial cells) and thus the mucus layer of the stomach offers it some degree of protection from the gastric juice. *H. pylori* is also capable of hydrolysing urea to ammonium via the action of a cell wall-bound urease, thereby creating a protective microenvironment [11] (Fig. 2).

The urease activity of *H. pylori* may be one of the major factors contributing to mucosal damage and inflammation seen in patients infected with this organism. *In vitro* experiments suggest that the ammonium ions produced by *H. pylori* are toxic to gastric epithelial cells. It is also possible that *H. pylori* releases other diffusible toxins that disrupt the gastric epithelium, although such factors have yet to be characterized. The observed presence of inflammatory cells beneath an intact epithelium in regions adjacent to *H. pylori* colonization suggests that some soluble factors with chemotactic properties may be released by the *H. pylori* and may gain access to the lamina propria (possibly an endotoxin, exotoxin or inflammatory mediator).

The links between *H. pylori* and gastritis, and between gastritis and duodenal ulcer are well established, yet the precise role of this micro-organism in the etiology of ulceration is

Table 2 **Risk factors associated with gastric or duodenal ulceration**

Substance	Proposed or known mechanism
NSAIDs	Inhibition of prostaglandin synthesis; direct cytotoxic effects
Ethanol	Vascular damage and stasis; direct cytotoxic effects
Smoking	Unknown; possibly decreases gastric prostaglandin synthesis and increases acid secretion
Corticosteroids	Inhibition of repair of pre-existing damage; interfere with acute inflammatory responses
Methylxanthines	Stimulation of acid secretion
Shock/trauma/burns	Decreased blood flow; circulating 'ulcerogenic' mediators of unknown nature or origin
H. pylori	Mucosal damage by ammonium ions, unidentified cytotoxins

Concentrations of ethanol in the range found in beer and wine (i.e. 4–15%) also stimulate gastric acid secretion; methylxanthines include caffeine and theophylline.

yet to be clearly defined. Although the incidence of *H. pylori* infection is very high in both gastric and duodenal ulceration, many individuals that test positive for the bacterium never develop ulcers. Duodenal ulceration is more common in males, but *H. pylori* is detected to equal degrees in both sexes. Moreover, ulcers can be healed by treatment with drugs that inhibit acid secretion, despite the continued presence in the stomach of *H. pylori.*

Only recently have clinical studies aimed at eradicating *H. pylori* infection with antimicrobials begun to more fully assess its role in ulceration and ulcer relapse. Antibiotic treatment, in combination with acid suppression, has proven to be much more effective at preventing ulcer relapse than acid suppression alone [12]. In fact, treatment with a combination of antibiotics and colloidal bismuth (which in some experimental conditions is also capable of killing *H. pylori*) was shown recently to prevent ulcer relapse for at least 12 months. Preparations of bismuth have been used in the treatment of gastric ulcer for over a century, but it is only the recent discovery of its effects on *H. pylori* that has provided information on how these preparations may exert their beneficial actions.

Non-steroidal anti-inflammatory drugs

A subset of ulcer disease which does not correlate with *H. pylori* colonization of the stomach is that associated with the use of non-steroidal anti-inflammatory drugs (NSAIDs; e.g. aspirin, indomethacin and ibuprofen). These drugs are used most commonly for treatment of joint inflammation (i.e. rheumatoid arthritis and osteoarthritis). It is estimated that approximately 20% of individuals taking NSAIDs over an extended period will develop a gastric ulcer [10]. This type of ulcer is most prevalent in elderly women and a particularly disturbing feature is that the ulcers are frequently 'silent'; that is, the patient does not exhibit symptoms or feel any pain. As a result, these patients often present at the hospital with a major haemorrhage or even with a perforated ulcer. Perforation of gastro-intestinal ulcers frequently leads to death.

While the pathogenesis of NSAID-induced ulceration is not fully understood, it appears that an important contributing factor is the ability of these drugs to inhibit gastric prostaglandin synthesis [13–15]. Prostaglandins are believed to play an important physiological role in modulating the various components of mucosal defence. For example, they stimulate the secretion of mucus and bicarbonate by the gastric and duodenal mucosae and play an important role in the reactive hyperaemic response to injury and acid back-diffusion. The ability of a NSAID to induce ulcers in experimental animals has been shown to correlate very well with the ability of

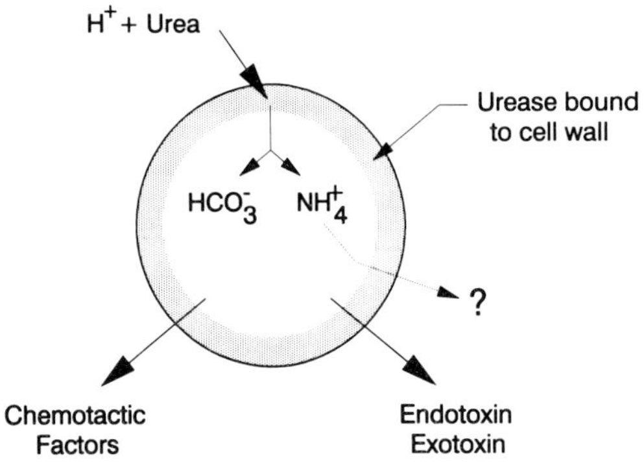

Fig. 2. Schematic diagram representing the mechanism by which *H. pylori* resists destruction by gastric acid, and some possible mechanisms by which it might produce epithelial damage in the stomach and duodenum

Cell wall-bound urease can catalyse the conversion of acid and urea to ammonium and bicarbonate. This bicarbonate may be important for allowing the bacterium to maintain an intracellular pH in the normal range and may also be secreted such that an external microenvironment of high pH is created. Urease itself may be capable of causing damage to epithelial cells, and may also have some chemotactic actions, resulting in the recruitment of inflammatory cells into the mucosa (other chemotactic factors may also be released by this organism). The ammonium produced through the urease activity may also contribute to the virulence of H. pylori. *This bacterium probably releases endotoxins or exotoxins which could contribute to the tissue damage and ulceration associated with colonization of the stomach or duodenum with this organism.*

that compound to inhibit gastric prostaglandin synthesis. Possibly through the reduction of mucosal prostaglandin synthesis, NSAIDs can reduce mucosal blood flow, thereby reducing the supply of oxygen and nutrients to the epithelium and reducing the ability of the mucosa to withstand exposure to toxins and endogenous irritants (e.g. acid). There is also experimental evidence suggesting that most NSAIDs have direct irritant effects on the gastric mucosa. NSAIDs are capable of inhibiting platelet aggregation, so that bleeding times are often prolonged in patients taking these drugs and bleeding from ulcers is frequently observed. In fact, patients with gastric or duodenal ulcers who are taking NSAIDs are three-times more likely to have clinically significant bleeds than ulcer patients not taking these drugs.

Alcohol

The ingestion of alcohol has long been known to cause damage to the gastric mucosa which occasionally is associated with significant bleeding. A link between the use of alcohol and peptic ulcer disease is less clear, at least in terms of alcohol actually causing gastric or duodenal ulcer. Certainly alcohol will exacerbate an existing ulcer.

Alcohol-induced gastric ulceration in the rat is probably the most frequently employed experimental model. Because of this, a great deal has been learned about the mechanism through which alcohol causes mucosal injury, and the mediators which might be involved in the process. Alcohol appears to cause mucosal injury through two distinct mechanisms [16]: firstly, by virtue of its lipophilic properties, it disrupts the surface epithelium in the stomach; and secondly, it causes vascular stasis. The epithelial injury produced by alcohol can usually be repaired rapidly through restitution. The vascular stasis is almost always accompanied by deeper mucosal ulceration. Healing of this type of damage requires several days. Considerable effort has been put into a search for a mediator responsible for the vasocongestion induced by alcohol. For example, it has been suggested that leukotrienes with vasoconstriction actions (e.g. LTC_4) may be released when the mucosa is exposed to alcohol, but there is no clear consensus on this issue [9]. Alcohol does not influence gastric prostaglandin synthesis, yet much of the damage induced by this substance can be prevented by pretreating the experimental animal with a prostaglandin. Prostaglandins reduce alcohol-induced injury most probably by preventing vascular stasis, although the mechanism responsible for this action has not yet been clearly identified.

Shock

Gastro-intestinal ulceration is frequently encountered in patients suffering from various forms of shock (e.g. endotoxic, haemorrhagic, hypotensive). Experimental evidence points to two major mechanisms through which shock can predispose a patient to ulceration. Firstly, the hypotension which accompanies shock results in reduced blood flow through the splanchnic circulation, since blood is redirected to 'vital' organs such as the heart and brain. Reduced blood flow renders the mucosa more susceptible to ulceration as the epithelium is deprived of oxygen and nutrients, and back-diffusing acid or toxins are permitted to accumulate. Secondly, a number of mediators are released in shock conditions which have been shown to produce mucosal ulceration. For example, platelet-activating factor and tumour necrosis factor have been shown to be released by macrophages when stimulated by endotoxin. These mediators can themselves induce hypotension and gastro-intestinal ulceration in experimental animals when administered systemically [17]. The precise mechanism through which they act is not yet fully understood.

Drugs used in the treatment of ulcer disease

Since ulceration of the stomach and duodenum occurs because of an imbalance between the aggressive factors present in the lumen and the mucosal defence system, treatment of these diseases could be targeted either at reducing the levels of aggressive factors or at enhancing mucosal defence. Virtually all of the treatment modalities presently employed are targeted at the former. For example, the most commonly prescribed drugs for the treatment of ulcer disease act through reduction of gastric acidity (Table 3). These include the antacids which neutralize existing acid, and a number of drugs which inhibit the secretion of acid. Histamine H_2 receptor antagonists (e.g. cimetidine, ranitidine), muscarinic receptor antagonists (e.g. pirenzipine) and H^+,K^+-ATPase (proton pump) inhibitors (e.g. omeprazole) all inhibit the secretion of acid from parietal (oxyntic) cells. By removing or reducing acid, repair can occur more rapidly. However, recurrence rates of gastro-intestinal ulceration one year after cessation of therapy approach 80%.

Prostaglandins, although having numerous effects on mucosal defence, appear to work clinically through their ability to inhibit acid secretion. Doses of prostaglandins which are below those necessary for inhibition of acid secretion have proven to be ineffective in the treatment of peptic ulcer disease. In the case of

Table 3 **Examples of treatments for peptic ulcer disease and the mechanisms of action**

Treatment	Proposed or known mechanism of action
H_2 receptor agonists (e.g. cimetidine, ranitidine)	Inhibition of acid secretion
H^+/K^+-ATPase inhibitors (e.g. omeprazole)	Inhibition of acid production
M receptor antagonist (e.g. pirenzipine)	Inhibition of acid secretion
Prostaglandin analogues (e.g. misoprostol)	Inhibition of acid secretion; direct 'cytoprotection' (mucus, HCO_3^- stimulation)
Sucralfate	Stimulation of prostaglandin synthesis; 'protection' of ulcer base; others?
Bismuth salts (e.g. De-NOL)	Eradication of *H. pylori*
Carbenoxolone	Stimulation of prostaglandin synthesis; inhibition of pepsin secretion
Antimicrobials (e.g. amoxycillin)	Eradication of *H. pylori*

Abbreviations used: H_2, histamine$_2$ receptor; M, muscarinic cholinergic receptor.

NSAID-induced gastropathy, prostaglandins appear to be the most effective therapeutic agents [10].

Carbenoxolone (a liquorice derivative) enjoyed some popularity, particularly in Europe, in the 1960s and 1970s, but is used less commonly now. The mechanism of action of this drug has never been clearly elucidated, but it has been suggested that it inhibits peptic activity and pepsin secretion, as well as stimulating endogenous prostaglandin synthesis.

Sucralfate is another drug used for treatment of gastro-duodenal ulceration with a poorly understood mechanism of action. This aluminium salt of sucrose octasulfate appears to bind to the ulcer base and, in some unknown way, promote healing. It has also been shown to stimulate prostaglandin synthesis in some experimental settings, which may contribute to its beneficial actions.

In recent years, bismuth salts and antimicrobials (e.g. amoxycillin, metronidazole) have been carefully evaluated in peptic ulcer patients. These agents are capable of accelerating the healing of ulcers and, perhaps more importantly, of preventing the relapse of ulcers. This latter effect occurs only if *H. pylori* is completely eradicated during the course of therapy with the agents [12].

Conclusions

▶ Significant advances have been made in recent years in terms of our understanding of the etiology and pathogenesis of ulcer disease.

▶ It is now clear that a large fraction of ulcer disease is directly related to colonization of the upper gastro-intestinal tract by the bacterium *H. pylori*, although the mechanisms through which this organism induces inflammation and ulceration are not yet clear.

▶ Another subset of ulcer disease, which is unrelated to *H. pylori*, is that associated with the use of NSAIDs; again, the pathogenesis of this type of ulcer is not fully understood.

▶ Alcohol consumption and various types of cardiovascular shock are further factors inducing gastric ulceration.

▶ Treatments include the administration of drugs that reduce gastric acid secretion (e.g. H_2 receptor antagonists) or stimulate mucus and bicarbonate secretion (e.g. prostaglandin analogues), or the eradication of *H. pylori.*

▶ Perhaps the greatest advances in this field during the past two decades have been in the elucidation of the various components of mucosal defence: since it appears that there must be a failure of mucosal defence for ulceration to occur, it is likely that a greater understanding of how the mucosa resists injury may lead to the elucidation of the pathogenesis of the various types of ulcer disease.

▶ Ultimately, a clearer understanding of the pathogenesis of ulcer disease will allow for the development of safer, more specific and effective therapies for these maladies.

References

1. Garner, A. and O'Brien, P. E. (1991) Mechanisms of injury, protection and repair of the upper gastrointestinal tract, p. 540, J. Wiley and Sons, Chichester
2. Wallace, J. L. (1990) Mucosal defence: new avenues for treatment of ulcer disease? In Gastroenterology Clinics of North America, Vol. 19 (Hunt, R. H., ed.), pp. 87–100, W. B. Saunders, Philadelphia
3. Allen, A. and Garner, A. (1980) Mucus and bicarbonate secretion in the stomach and their possible role in mucosal protection. Gut **21**, 249–262
4. Silen, W. and Ito, S. (1985) Mechanisms for rapid re-epithelialization of the gastric mucosal surface. Annu. Rev. Physiol. **47**, 217–229
5. Morris, G. P. (1986) The myth of the mucus barrier. Gastroenterol. Clin. Biol. **12**, 106–107
6. Wallace, J. L. and Whittle, B. J. R. (1986) Role of mucus in repair of epithelial damage in the rat. Inhibition of epithelial recovery by mucolytic agents. Gastroenterology **91**, 603–611
7. Hawkey, C. J. and Rampton, D. S. (1985) Prostaglandins and the gastrointestinal mucosa: are they important in its function, disease, or treatment? Gastroenterology **89**, 1162–1188
8. Whittle, B. J. R. (1977) Mechanisms underlying gastric mucosal damage induced by indomethacin and bile salts, and the actions of prostaglandins. Br. J. Pharmacol. **60**, 455–460
9. Wallace, J. L. (1990) Lipid mediators of inflammation in gastric ulcer. Am. J. Physiol. **258**, G1–G11
10. Graham, D. Y. (1990) The relationship between non-steroidal anti-inflammatory drug use and peptic ulcer disease. In Gastroenterology Clinics of North America, Vol. 19 (Hunt, R. H., ed.), pp. 171–182, W. B. Saunders, Philadelphia
11. Marshall, B. J., Barrett, L. J., Prakash, C., McCallum, R. W. and Guerrant, R. L. (1990) Urea protects *Helicobacter* (*Campylobacter*) *pylori* from the bactericidal effect of acid. Gastroenterology **99**, 697–702
12. Rauws, E. A. J. and Tytgat, G. N. J. (1990) Cure of duodenal ulcer associated with eradication of *Helicobacter pylori*. Lancet **335**, 1233–1235
13. Whittle, B. J. R. (1981) Temporal relationship between cycloxygenase inhibition, as measured by prostacyclin biosynthesis, and the gastrointestinal damage induced by indomethacin in the rat. Gastroenterology **80**, 94–98

14. Hawkey, C. J. (1989) Prostaglandins and mucosal protection: laboratory evidence versus clinical performance. In Advances in Drug Therapy of Gastrointestinal Ulceration (Garner, A. and Whittle, B. J. R., eds.), pp. 89–107, J. Wiley and Sons, Chichester
15. Soll, A. H. (1991 Non-steroidal anti-inflammatory drugs and peptic ulcer disease. Anim. Internal Med. **114**, 307–319
16. Oates, P. J. and Hakkinen, J. P. (1988) Studies on the mechanism of ethanol-induced gastric damage in rats. Gastroenterology **94**, 10–21
17. Espluges, J. V., Whittle, B. J. R. and Moncada, S. C. (1989) Local opioid-sensitive afferent sensory neurones in the modulation of gastric damage induced by PAF. Br. J. Pharmacol. **97**, 579–585

10

Coughing: an airway defensive reflex

Giuseppe Sant'Ambrogio
Department of Physiology and Biophysics, University of Texas Medical Branch, Galveston, TX 77550, U.S.A.

Introduction

Cough constitutes a defence mechanism that protects the lungs against aspiration of foreign material and removes excessive airway (mostly tracheobronchial) secretions. Coughing is recognizable by its characteristic sound; indeed the word cough has a clear onomatopoeic connotation since it reproduces the sound associated with it.

Cough involves the activation of several muscles, all having a prevalent respiratory function, that act on either the chest wall or the upper airway. These muscles become activated sequentially with a well co-ordinated and fixed pattern that has suggested the presence of a separate and specialized neural centre. Indeed, even the descending motor pathways implicated in the act of coughing can be controlled independently from their actions in normal breathing.

The act of coughing occurs in three successive phases. In the first 'inspiratory phase' a volume of air larger than tidal volume at rest is drawn into the lungs. During the following 'compressive phase' the glottis is shut while thoracic and abdominal expiratory muscles contract forcefully. A sudden decompression takes place in the subsequent 'expulsive phase' as the glottis is opened and a blast of air is blown out at a very high flow rate. Coryllos [1] compared the three phases of coughing to the three phases of the deflagration of a gun: the inspiratory phase to the loading of the gun, the compressive phase to the deflagration of powder and production of gases under pressure, and the expulsive phase to the ejection of the bullet from the barrel of the gun. Fig. 1 depicts schematically the acoustic, geometric, mechanical and electromyographic

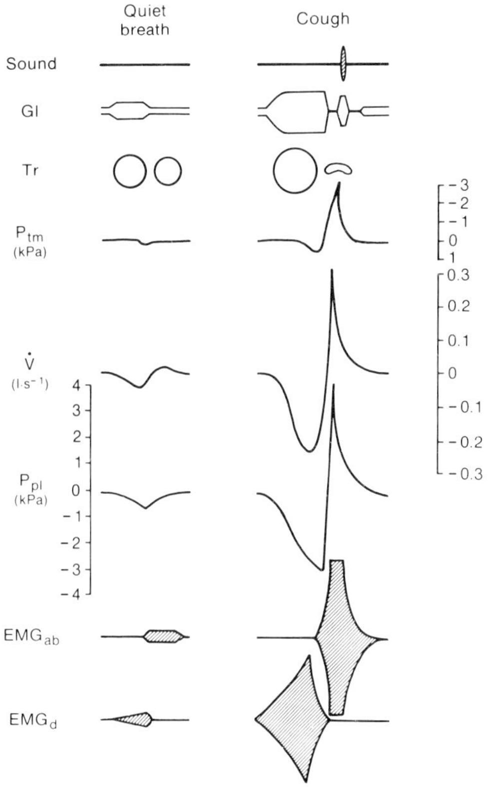

Fig. 1. The acoustic, geometric, mechanical and electromyographic events in cough and quiet breath

Shown here are the changes in cough sound, glottal (G1) and tracheal (Tr) cross-sectional areas, transmural pressure [P_{tm}; kPa (scale on right)] at the level of large airways, airflow [$\dot{V}$, $l\ s^{-1}$ (scale on right)], intrathoracic pressure (P_{pl}; kPa), abdominal (EMG_{ab}) and diaphragmatic (EMG_d) electromyograms. Modified from [13].

events that occur in cough, compared with those of a quiet breath.

Coughing does not normally occur in healthy individuals, although they can cough in response to exogenous mechanical and chemical irritants. In these circumstances cough intervenes as a supplemental mechanism to the mucociliary escalator in response to the irritant stimulus itself or to the excessive secretion that has overloaded the ciliary function. Cough is a very frequent and important symptom of many respiratory diseases in which it is triggered by endogenous stimuli such as mucus hypersecretion, mucosal swelling, epithelial sloughing and increase in epithelial permeability.

The effectiveness of coughing as a clearance mechanism for the tracheobronchial tree depends on (i) the presence of a sufficiently thick mucus layer lining the airway mucosa and (ii) the linear velocity of the air flowing through the airway in an expiratory direction.

Mucus production and cough

The importance of the mucus layer has been demonstrated clearly in bronchitic patients with an impaired mucociliary clearance but an abundant mucus secretion [2]. In fact, these patients could achieve normal clearance rates when they coughed. On the other hand, voluntary coughing in healthy individuals has no effect on clearance rates. It is interesting to note that irritant stimuli capable of eliciting cough are also effective in promoting mucus secretion, presumably acting through the same afferent pathway.

Mechanics of cough

The other factor that determines the effectiveness of cough depends upon the velocity at which air flows through the airway; this depends on the cross-sectional area of the airway as follows:

$$\text{Velocity} = \frac{\text{Air flow rate}}{\text{Cross-sectional area}}$$

Considering the geometry of the tracheobronchial airway we see that the total cross-sectional area becomes progressively smaller moving from the alveolar space towards the larynx. This means that, for a given volume of air, linear velocity of flow must in general be higher in large airways than in small airways. Furthermore, activation of expiratory muscles during the compressive phase of cough renders intrapleural pressure greater than atmospheric pressure. Alveolar pressure, due to the elastic recoil of the lungs, will be even greater than pleural pressure. As the glottis is opened during the expulsive phase, pressure at the airway opening (mouth) remains atmospheric while pressure in the airways at the alveolar end is still greater than pleural pressure keeping the airway distended. Since pleural pressure is approximately equal throughout the thoracic cavity, i.e. on the outside of all intrathoracic airways, and intraluminal pressure decreases from the alveolar end toward the airway opening, there must be a point along the airway where pleural and intraluminal pressures are equal (equal pressure point; EPP). Upstream from this point (i.e. toward the alveoli), airways are distended, while downstream from this point airways are compressed. Indeed, during coughing the cross-sectional areas of the trachea and the main bronchi undergo considerable narrowings with corresponding increases in linear velocities of the expired air that improve the scrubbing action of coughing (Fig. 2) [3].

Coughing usually occurs as a succession of interrupted expirations starting after a deep inspiration and ending at residual volume. This pattern of coughing probably provides a better clearing mechanism than a single forced expiration. In fact the presence of a series of rapidly changing transmural pressure swings acting on the walls of the airways would help to loosen the mucus accumulated on the mucosal surface.

Coughing can be performed voluntarily, but in most circumstances is a reflex response elicited primarily by irritant stimuli to the larynx and the tracheobronchial tree. Cough is uniquely dependent on vagal afferents [4]; even extrarespiratory sources of cough, like the tympanic membrane and the external auditory meatus [5], are supplied by vagal afferents of the auricular nerve.

Cough and bronchoconstriction

Cough and bronchoconstriction are often associated, but they can generally be recognized as

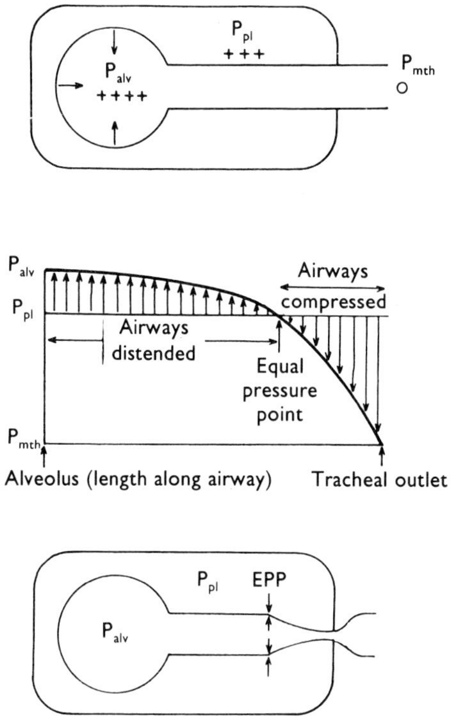

Fig. 2. Mechanics of cough
The upper panel shows a model of lungs during cough. Where pleural pressure (P_{pl}) is greater than atmospheric, pressure in the alveoli (P_{alv}) is greater than P_{pl} because of the elastic recoil of the lung (arrows), and mouth pressure is atmospheric. Because P_{pl} is approximately the pressure acting on the outer wall of the airways, the pressure in the airways at the alveolar end is greater than the pressure outside them. The opposite is the case at the mouth end. Thus, there must be points along the airway where intraluminal pressures equal pleural pressures (equal pressure points, EPPs). Compression of the airways occurs between an EPP and the thoracic outlet (lower panel). The pressure inter-relationships are shown diagrammatically in the middle panel which plots a hypothetical pressure drop from the alveolus (P_{alv}) to the tracheal outlet within the airways (curved line). The pressure outside the airways (P_{pl}) is given by the horizontal line. EPPs are shown where the two lines intersect. Between EPP and alveoli the airways are distended (upward directed arrows). Between EPP and the tracheal outlet the airways are compressed (downward directed arrows). Reproduced from [3] with permission.

separate mechanisms. They can be induced separately and can be differentially inhibited by drugs. For instance, inhalation of nebulized water is a well recognized stimulus for eliciting both cough and bronchoconstriction. However, whereas cough depends on a lack of permeant anions (e.g. chloride, which can diffuse into the mucosa), bronchoconstriction depends on the tonicity of the solution [6]. In addition, the variable effects of bronchodilating drugs on cough suggest that airway tone has little influence on the responsiveness to tussive agents. In any event, it is clear that bronchomotor tone can be altered by inputs that do not elicit cough, e.g. chemoreceptor stimulation, contraction of skeletal muscles and irritation of the nose and nasopharynx. Spontaneous cough is strictly a reflex mediated by the central nervous system, and bronchoconstriction, although often mediated in the same manner, may also be elicited by the release of mediators from afferent nerve fibres.

Cough, sleep and anaesthesia

An important characteristic of the cough reflex is its strong dependency on the sleep–wakefulness state. In fact, coughing in response to mechanical and chemical irritation of the larynx and tracheobronchial airways is found to be strictly linked to arousal [7, 8]. A stimulus (e.g. inhalation of a small balloon in the laryngeal lumen, squirting a small volume of water into the larynx or trachea, inhalation of acetic acid through a tracheostomy) capable of eliciting cough in dogs during wakefulness becomes ineffective during either slow wave (SWS) or rapid eye movement (REM) sleep. Only when the stimulus intensity is sufficient to cause arousal does cough occur, and it always follows arousal. The intensity of laryngeal or tracheobronchial stimulation necessary to produce arousal and coughing is higher in REM than SWS. As noted by Sullivan et al. [7, 8], since other reflex effects of laryngeal stimulation (expiration reflex, apnoea and bradycardia) can be elicited without arousal, the absence of the cough reflex cannot be attributed to a diminished function of airway receptors during sleep. These observations rather suggest that the act of coughing, at variance with normal breathing, relies on supramedullary neural processes normally functioning only during wakefulness.

A similar situation is seen in patients under anaesthesia, the level of anaesthesia having a marked influence on the reflex responses to airway irritation. Experiments conducted by Nishino and co-workers [9] on human subjects under different levels of enflurane anaesthetic provide a good example. Upon instillation of a small volume of water (1.0 ml) into the trachea under the highest enflurane level used [1.3 minimum alveolar concentration (MAC)], none of the patients coughed; the most frequent response was instead a prompt apnoea. The cough reflex was present, however, in 23% of the patients at 1.0 MAC and in 69% of the patients at 0.7 MAC. On the other hand, the apnoeic response showed an opposite trend, becoming less frequent at lighter anaesthetic levels.

▶ Cough is usually a reflex response elicited by irritant stimuli to the larynx and tracheobronchial tree; it consists of inspiratory, compressive and expulsive phases.
▶ Two factors affecting the effectiveness of cough are the presence of mucus and the velocity at which air flows through the airway.
▶ Although cough and bronchoconstriction are often associated, they can be recognized, by their respective means of induction, as two separate mechanisms.
▶ The cough reflex cannot be elicited during sleep without arousal, nor during anaesthesia.

Neurology of cough

Inhalation of various irritants and particulate matter can trigger several reflex responses, cough being one of them. The concentration of irritants is likely to be higher at the level of the pharynx and larynx and to decrease toward the periphery of the lungs. This implies a strong stimulation of receptors in the larynx which, in fact, together with the points of branching of the more proximal subdivisions of the tracheobronchial tree, is particularly responsive to tussigenic stimuli. The tussigenic areas coincide, at least in some species, with regions with a high density of free nerve endings within and just beneath the airway epithelium [4, 10]. Because of the marked differences in morphology and afferent input, the two main tussigenic sites — larynx and tracheobronchial tree — will be discussed separately.

The larynx

The main source of afferent fibres to the larynx is the internal branch of the superior laryngeal nerve. Recordings from the peripheral cut-end of this nerve in animals breathing through their upper airway show the presence of a marked respiratory modulation. This respiratory-related activity is controlled by afferent endings activated by the inspiratory cooling of the laryngeal lumen (cold receptors), pressure-responsive receptors, and receptors stimulated by the contracting intrinsic laryngeal muscles and the tracheal tug [11]. Besides these afferent modalities closely related to respiratory events, there is another type of laryngeal afferent, scarcely active in control conditions but readily stimulated by various mechanical and chemical irritants known for their tussigenic properties (Fig. 3). These 'irritant' type receptors have myelinated fibres, and a large proportion respond with a rapid increase in activity to administration of water or water solutions lacking chloride ions, two stimuli also known to induce cough in most subjects [12]. All things considered it seems reasonable to conclude that the stimulation of these 'irritant' receptors with myelinated fibres is responsible for laryngeal cough.

However, an exclusive role for myelinated afferents in cough from the larynx is not supported by the observation that cough can also be provoked by inhalation of capsaicin, supposedly a selective stimulant of C-fibre endings. At least in humans the tussigenic effect of aerosolized capsaicin can be blocked by laryngeal anaesthesia. These results imply a role for C-fibre receptors in the cough elicited from the larynx.

According to Korpas and Tomori [13], cough elicited from the larynx shows some distinctive features compared with that from the tracheobronchial tree. The inspiratory phase is more pronounced while the expiratory phase is less pronounced and the frequency of the expiratory efforts much higher. Laryngeal cough is also less susceptible to drugs and to conditions such as hypothermia and hyperthermia.

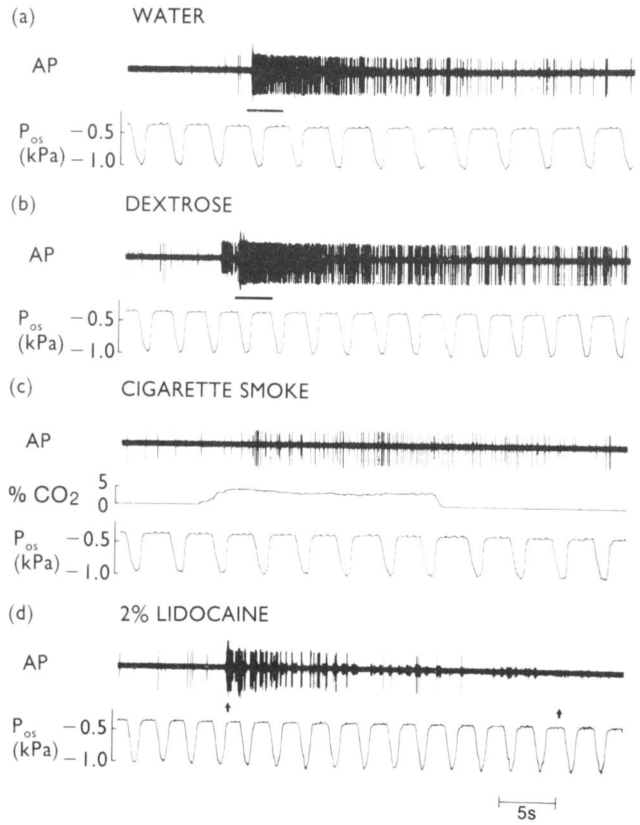

Fig. 3. Response of a laryngeal 'irritant' receptor to known tussigenic stimuli

Note the prompt and vigorous activation of the receptor elicited by both water and isosmotic dextrose (**a,b**)*. This indicates that lack of chloride anions, rather than osmolarity, is causing the receptor discharge. Exposure of the upper airway to smoke* (**c**) *is indicated by the CO_2 signal. The response of the receptor to mechanical stimulation* (**d**) *was abolished by lidocaine in 21 s. This stimulation was performed (between arrows) with a cotton applicator soaked in a 2% (w/v) solution of lidocaine. The relatively short blocking time of 2% lidocaine indicates a superficial location of this receptor. Abbreviations used: AP, action potential; P_{os}, oesophageal pressure.*

The tracheobronchial tree

Cough can readily be elicited by irritant stimuli delivered to the tracheobronchial tree. It is generally agreed that the more peripheral bronchial branches are less important as tussigenic sites. Vagal afferents have been found consistently to be essential for the elicitation of cough from the tracheobronchial airways (Fig. 4) [13]. Cough from one side of the bronchial tree can be abolished by ipsilateral vagotomy [14].

All four types of receptors (slowly adapting stretch receptors, rapidly adapting receptors, bronchial and pulmonary C-fibre receptors) described as present within the tracheobronchial tree and the lung parenchyma have been implicated in the cough reflex. Opinions differ among investigators concerning the relative roles of the different receptor types; particularly disputed is the role of C-fibre endings. Strong evidence supports an important role for myelinated vagal afferents in tracheobronchial cough. A selective block of vagal conduction affecting mostly, although not exclusively, myelinated fibres, renders ineffective various tussigenic stimuli. Similarly, dogs in which acrylamide administration had induced a severe neuropathy with a selective

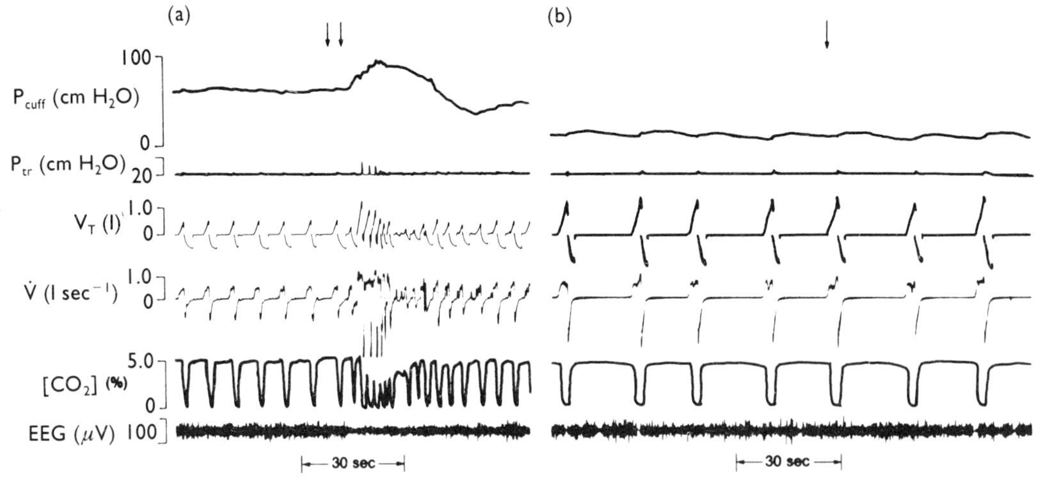

Fig. 4. Tracings showing the effect of bilateral vagal blockade on arousal and the ventilatory response to inhalation of acetic acid vapour

In the control recording (**a**), *inhalation of one breath of acetic acid vapour (1st arrow) during slow wave sleep caused arousal (2nd arrow), followed by coughing and reflex tracheal smooth muscle constriction. During slow wave sleep with bilateral vagal blockade* (**b**), *inhalation of one breath of the same vapour did not cause arousal, coughing or tracheal muscle contraction. Note the marked decrease in P_{cuff}, and hence the resting smooth muscle tone, during vagal blockade. Reproduced from [8] with permission. Abbreviations used: EEG, electroencephalogram; P_{cuff}, pressure within the cuff of an endotracheal tube indicating changes in bronchomotor tone; P_{tr}, tracheal pressure; $\dot{V}$, airflow, V_T, tidal volume.*

impairment of vagal myelinated fibres became unable to cough in response to irritants administered through a tracheostomy (M. I. Hersch, personal communication).

Rapidly adapting receptors

Several neurophysiological studies have demonstrated the presence in the more proximal areas of the tracheobronchial tree of a type of receptor, with myelinated fibres, that is strongly and promptly activated by well recognized tussigenic stimuli. These receptors, in consideration of their rate of adaptation to a mechanical stimulus, are defined as 'rapidly adapting receptors' (RAR) and for the kind of stimuli that can activate them as 'irritant receptors' [10]. They are most concentrated in the more proximal portions of the tracheobronchial tree, particularly at the points of branching, and have a superficial location within the airway mucosa. Their location coincides with the most sensitive tussigenic sites and is consistent with their ability to respond to light mechanical and weak chemical irritations. The lower occurrence of coughing in newborn animals and infants is also consistent with the scant RAR activity seen in the early stages of life [4].

Slowly adapting receptors

The view that slowly adapting receptors (SAR) may be implicated in coughing was proposed several years ago by Bucher [15], and has received some experimental support more recently. In fact, it was found that a selective block of SARs, obtainable in rabbits inhaling high concentrations of sulphur dioxide, can abolish the tussive response to mechanical and chemical irritant stimuli that, however, are still capable of activating rapidly adapting irritant receptors [16, 17]. Since SARs are not generally stimulated by known tussigenic irritants such as light mechanical probing of the extrapulmonary airways, it seems unlikely that they are directly involved in coughing. They could, however, play an indirect role by facilitating the reflex activation of expiratory muscles — an essential part of coughing.

Bronchial and pulmonary C-fibre receptors

Non-myelinated (C-fibre) afferents constitute the vast majority of vagal afferent fibres distributed to the tracheobronchial tree and the lung. For instance, in the bronchial vagal branches of the cat the ratio of non-myelinated to myelinated fibres is 11:1 [18]. C-fibre afferents are normally silent or have a sparse activity and are usually studied by eliciting their activity with extraneous substances like capsaicin and phenyl biguanide that are described as 'specific' or 'selective' stimulants of these endings. An important point to consider when evaluating the 'selectivity' of these substances is that they may be selective when used in 'threshold doses', but unselective when these doses are exceeded. With higher doses afferents with myelinated fibres may also be activated.

On the basis of their circulatory accessibility two types of C-fibre receptors have been described: 'pulmonary', which can be stimulated by a challenging drug more readily through the pulmonary circulation than the systemic circulation, and 'bronchial', which show a preferential accessibility through the systemic circulation.

The two categories of endings have different chemosensitivities to some naturally occurring substances. For instance, bradykinin, histamine, 5-hydroxytryptamine and prostaglandins (of the F and E series) stimulate bronchial C-fibre endings, whereas prostaglandin E_2 stimulates pulmonary C-fibre endings [19].

C-fibre endings play an important role in the regulation of airway smooth muscle tone and mucus secretion and also contribute toward the regulation of the breathing pattern.

Observations in man and experimental animals seem to support a significant role of C-fibre receptors in coughing. Exposure of unanaesthetized guinea pigs to nebulized solutions of capsaicin produces cough and sneezes as well as bronchoconstriction. Animals of the same species, pretreated with large doses of capsaicin that has a selective neurotoxic action on polymodal nociceptors predominantly constituted by C-fibre afferents, can still cough in response to mechanical irritation of the larynx and trachea as well as to inhalation of cigarette smoke (both capable of stimulating RARs), but are unresponsive to capsaicin. It thus seems that, in guinea pigs, the cough reflex can be mediated by both capsaicin-sensitive (C-fibres) and capsaicin-resistant (myelinated fibres) afferents [4].

Cough is readily elicited in humans inhaling nebulized solutions of capsaicin and also in one of three subjects who were given an intravenous low dose of capsaicin. Inhalation of a bradykinin aerosol at a concentration that activates bronchial C-fibres in dogs elicits cough in humans. Sulphur dioxide administered through a tracheostomy elicits cough in the dog, and at the same concentration activates C-fibre endings without much effect on SARs and RARs; the response is inhibited by cold (0–1°C) blocking the vagus nerves. Prostaglandin $F_{2\alpha}$, E_2 and E_1 inhaled as nebulized solutions produce cough, particularly in cats and humans. While $PGF_{2\alpha}$ activates both RARs and C-fibre receptors, PGE_1 and PGE_2 stimulate C-fibre endings only [4]. Cough is also a well recognized side-effect of angiotensin-converting enzyme inhibitors (e.g. captopril). The mechanisms of action of these inhibitors have been attributed to a decreased breakdown of bradykinin and substance P or to an increased production of prostaglandins. Any of these three mediators could then elicit cough, by stimulating C-fibre receptors.

Although the above evidence favours a role for C-fibre receptors as initiators of cough, other experimental results do not support this view. For instance, in experimental animals, either with or without anaesthesia, pulmonary C-fibre receptors, while mediating the so-called pulmonary chemoreflex (apnoea followed by rapid, shallow breathing, bradycardia and hypotension), do not induce coughing. It was actually found that in cats the stimulation of pulmonary C-fibre receptors has an inhibitory effect on the cough elicited from the larynx and tracheobronchial tree [20].

- ▶ Laryngeal cough is elicited by the stimulation of irritant receptors with myelinated fibres and C-fibre receptors; it is characterized by a more pronounced inspiratory phase and a less pronounced expiratory phase with more frequent expiratory efforts.
- ▶ Tracheobronchial cough involves four types of receptors present within the tracheobronchial tree.
- ▶ SARs play an indirect role in cough by facilitating the reflex activation of expiratory muscle.

▶ Pulmonary and bronchial non-myelinated C-fibre receptors are known to regulate airway smooth muscle tone, mucus secretion and breathing pattern, but whether they act as initiators of cough remains a controversy.

Conclusions

▶ Although the true reflex nature of cough — the involvement of vagal afferents, the central nervous system and the motor output to upper airway (abductors and adductor muscles) and chest wall muscles (inspiratory and expiratory) — is established, the identification of a particular type of receptor as the sole initiator of cough does not seem possible.

▶ Different stimuli can be equally effective in evoking cough and yet their respective efficacies to stimulate a certain type of receptor may be quite different.

▶ Perhaps the concept of one type of receptor involved only in one reflex response is too simplistic, and, more realistically, we should consider the possibility of different types of receptors contributing to a certain reflex response.

▶ A given pattern of motor response would correspond to a certain configuration of afferent input.

References

1. Coryllos, P. N. (1937) Action of the diaphragm in cough. Experimental and clinical study on the human. Amer. J. Med. Sci. **194**, 523–535
2. Camner, P., Mossberg, B. and Philipson, K. (1973) Tracheobronchial clearance in chronic obstructive lung disease. Scand. J. Resp. Dis. **54**, 272–281
3. Macklem, P. T. (1974) Physiology of cough. Ann. Otol. **83**, 761–768
4. Karlsson, J.-A., Sant'Ambrogio, G. and Widdicombe, J. G. (1988) Afferent neural pathways in cough and reflex bronchoconstriction. J. Appl. Physiol. **65**, 1007–1023
5. Todisco, T. (1982) The oto-respiratory reflex. Respiration **43**, 354–358
6. Eschenbacher, W. L., Boushey, H. A. and Shepard, D. (1984) Alteration in osmolarity of inhaled aerosols causes bronchial constriction and cough, but absence of a permeant anion causes cough alone. Am. Rev. Respir. Dis. **129**, 211–215
7. Sullivan, C. E., Murphy, L. F., Kozar, L. F. and Philipson, E. A. (1978) Waking and ventilatory responses to laryngeal stimulation in sleeping dogs. J. Appl. Physiol. **45**, 681–689
8. Sullivan, C. E., Kozar, L. F., Murphy, E. and Philipson, E. A. (1979) Arousal, ventilatory, and airway responses to bronchopulmonary stimulation in sleeping dogs. J. Appl. Physiol. **47**, 17–25
9. Nishino, T., Hiraga, K., Mizuguchi, T. and Honda, Y. (1988) Respiratory reflex responses to stimulation of tracheal mucosa in enflurane-anesthetized humans. J. Appl. Physiol. **65**, 1069–1074
10. Widdicombe, J. G. (1986) Sensory innervation of the lung and airways. In Progress in Brain Research. Visceral Sensations (Cervero, F. and Morrison, J. F. B., eds.), pp. 49–64, Elsevier, Amsterdam
11. Sant'Ambrogio, G., Mathew, O. P., Fisher, J. T. and Sant'Ambrogio, F. B. (1983) Laryngeal receptors responding to transmural pressure, airflow and local muscle activity. Respir. Physiol. **54**, 317–333
12. Anderson, J. W., Sant'Ambrogio, F. B., Mathew, O. P. and Sant'Ambrogio, G. (1990) Water responsive laryngeal receptors in the dog are not specialized endings. Respir. Physiol. **79**, 33–44
13. Korpas. J. and Tomori, Z. (1979) Cough and Other Respiratory Reflexes, Karger, Basel
14. Klassen, K. P., Morton, D. R. and Curtis, G. M. (1951) The clinical physiology of the human bronchi. III. The effect of vagus section on the cough reflex, bronchial caliber and clearance of bronchial secretions. Surgery **29**, 483–490
15. Bucher, K. (1958) Pathophysiology of cough. Pharmacol. Rev. **10**, 43–58
16. Sant'Ambrogio, G., Sant'Ambrogio, F. B. and Davies, A. (1984) Airway receptors in cough. Bull. Eur. Physiopathol. Respir. **20**, 43–47
17. Hanacek, J., Davies, A. and Widdicombe, J. G. (1984) Influence of lung stretch receptors on the cough reflex in rabbits. Respiration **45**, 161–168
18. Jammes, Y., Fornaris, E., Mei, S. S. and Barrat, E. (1982) Afferent and efferent components of the bronchial vagal branches in cats. J. Auton. Nerv. Syst. **5**, 165–176
19. Coleridge, J. C. M. and Coleridge, H. M. (1984) Afferent vagal C-fiber innervation of the lungs and airways and its functional significance. Rev. Physiol. Biochem. Pharmacol. **99**, 1–110
20. Tatar, M., Webber, S. E. and Widdicombe, J. G. (1988) Lung C-fibre receptor activation and defensive reflexes in anaesthetized cats. J. Physiol. **402**, 411–420

11

Vomiting: a gastro-intestinal tract defensive reflex

Paul Andrews
Department of Physiology, St George's Hospital Medical School, Cranmer Terrace, Tooting, London SW17 0RE, U.K.

Nausea and vomiting as defensive reflexes

In the essential functions of eating and drinking the body exposes itself to toxins. Usually efforts are made to avoid ingestion of potentially hazardous agents by taking evasive action as a result of visual, gustatory and olfactory inputs as poisonous animals and plants are often brightly coloured, bitter tasting or foul smelling. These senses may be regarded as the first level of defence against accidental poisoning. If ingestion of potential toxins cannot be avoided because the toxin is colourless, odourless or tasteless or simply because it is masked by the food itself, then its presence in the body must be detected rapidly. The detectors in the gut (pre-absorptive) and circulation (post-absorptive) trigger a series of events which confine the food to the stomach or limit further absorption and lead to its eventual ejection by vomiting itself. The levels of defence are summarized in Fig. 1 and will be discussed further later on.

In many respects the vomiting reflex has a similar function in the gut to the sneezing and cough reflexes in the respiratory system (see Chapter 10).

The survival value of having a system to eject poisons from the body is self-evident and the vomiting reflex has been demonstrated in members of many vertebrate classes: primates (e.g. man and squirrel monkey), carnivores (e.g. cat, dog and ferret), ruminants (e.g. sheep), birds (e.g. pigeon), reptiles (e.g. alligator), amphibia (e.g. frog) and fishes (e.g. shark, trout and tuna).

It could be argued that the vomiting reflex is of only minor significance in Western society with modern methods of food storage and preparation. However, it is estimated that there may be one million cases of food poisoning in the UK annually. (Source: *The Independent* newspaper, 23rd March 1991). A survey of students revealed that, while alcohol (a self-administered poison!) was the commonest cause of vomiting, some 15% reported that they had vomited at least once in the previous year as a result of what they thought was contaminated food. Obviously this reflex still has survival value. In addition to actual ejection of the toxin, the vomiting and the nausea which usually accompanies it are important in that they indicate to the animal that it has eaten contaminated food which should be avoided in the future.

Why do some species not have a vomiting reflex?

In spite of the obvious importance of vomiting, major mammalian groups such as rodents (e.g. rats and mice) and lagomorphs (rabbits) do not vomit. They do appear to exhibit behaviour which may be indicative of nausea, however. So how do such animals cope with poisons in the diet? We do not know the answer to this question with any degree of certainty but several different strategies can be demonstrated in animals without a vomiting reflex.

(i) In the rat, the sense of taste is acute and conditioned taste aversion is developed readily. Thus, if the animal ingests a food which makes it feel nauseated, it will form a memory linking the taste of the food and the malaise. When that taste is encountered again the animal will reject the food after only a few licks. It is this behaviour (bait-shyness) that makes rats so hard to kill by poisoning. This form of operant conditioning also occurs in humans. It is particularly potent if the memory is formed in

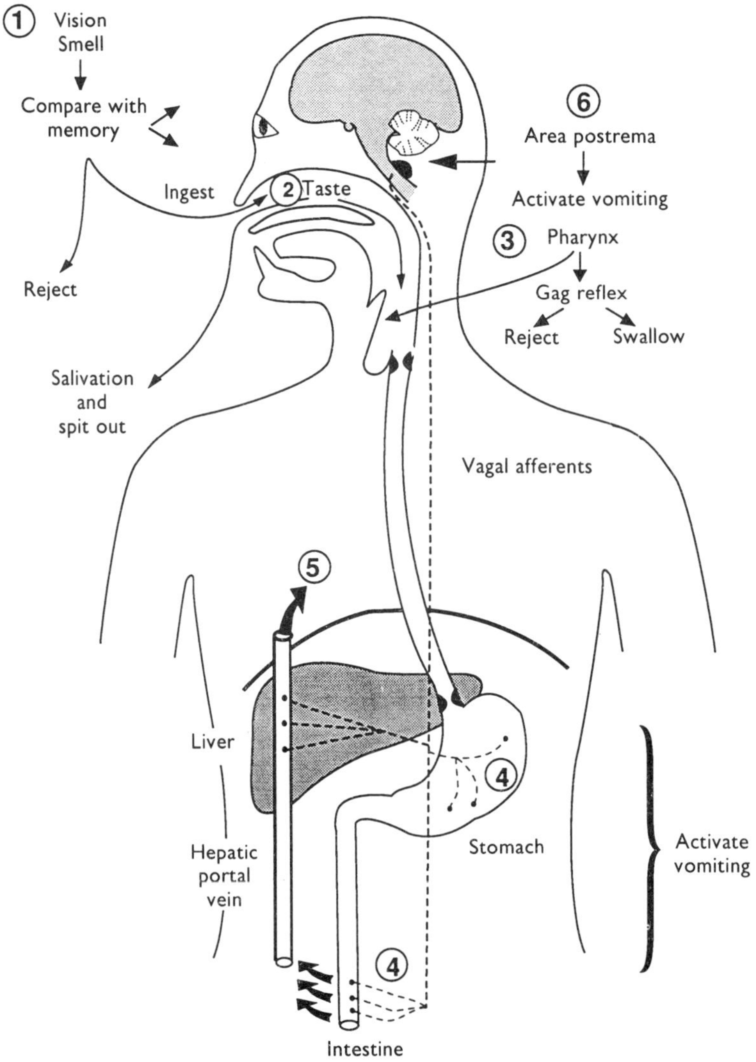

Fig. 1. A summary of the levels of defence employed against the ingestion of potential toxins in the diet.

early childhood and some researchers claim that nausea is a more potent aversive stimulus than pain in man [1]. Indeed, use has been made of conditioned taste aversion in the treatment of chronic alcoholics by coupling the presentation of alcohol with the administration of an emetic (vomit-inducing) agent.

(ii) Some animals eat foods containing poisons, presumably to allow them to exploit a food source not available to many other species. For example the koala bear eats eucalyptus leaves which may contain concentrations of prussic acid fatal to other species. However, its intestinal flora can detoxify the leaves. A different strategy is adopted by scarlet macaws. They eat soil containing kaolin which adsorbs the poisons contained in the seeds they eat at certain times of year. Poisoned rats also exhibit this behaviour.

Although we have focused on vomiting as a means of ejecting toxins rapidly from the body, the diarrhoea which often accompanies food poisoning may have a similar role.

Vomiting in a clinical context

From the above sections it can be seen that nausea and vomiting are components of the body's defensive system against ingested poisons and it is important to bear this in mind when considering the mechanisms by which vomiting is induced in clinical situations.

In general, nausea and vomiting are encountered clinically either as symptoms of a bewildering range of diseases (Table 1) or as side effects of therapeutic interventions including drug administration (e.g. anti-cancer cytotoxic drugs) and surgery (e.g. truncal vagotomy). Vomiting may be induced deliberately using apomorphine (see below) or ipecacuanha syrup as a treatment for self-administered poisoning.

Looking at the list of stimuli which induce vomiting they appear to have little in common. However, if we use the criterion of whether the vomiting leads to removal of the emetic stimulus it is possible to identify two groups:

— 'appropriate vomiting' where the stimulus is ejected from the body
— 'inappropriate vomiting' where the act of vomiting does not get rid of the stimulus.

On this basis the only 'appropriate vomiting' is that induced by stimuli arriving by the oral (natural) route or clinical conditions in which the upper gut becomes overdistended (e.g. gastric stasis). In these cases vomiting leads to the removal of the stimulus responsible for its induction. Most other forms of vomiting appear to be 'inappropriate'. For example, vomiting induced by drugs given intravenously, by motion or by pregnancy does not lead to removal of the emetic stimulus. The motor components of vomiting induced by the two groups of stimuli appear to be identical. For the 'inappropriate' stimuli to induce vomiting all that is required is that they activate receptors and pathways which are there for the detection of 'appropriate' stimuli. Thus, it is not necessary to postulate unique mechanisms for each clinical emetic stimulus but only to bear in mind that they probably act via pathways present for the detection of orally ingested poisons.

With these considerations in mind, the motor components of the vomiting reflex will be discussed together with the central integrative mechanisms and afferent inputs.

Table 1 **Examples of stimuli evoking the vomiting reflex**

Natural	Clinical	
	Therapeutic	Disease
Animal toxins, e.g. snake bite	Cytotoxic chemotherapy drugs	Addisons disease
		Diabetic gastroparesis
Food poisoning	Oral L-dopa	Diabetic ketoacidosis
Motion	Surgery and anaesthesia	Familial dysautonomia
Pregnancy	Morphine	Hepatitis
		Hypercalcaemia
		Hypertrophic pyloric stenosis
		Intestinal obstruction
		Labyrynthitis
		Medullary lesions e.g. Wallenberg syndrome
		Mesenteric ischaemia
		Pancreatitis
		Psychiatric disorders
		Raised intracranial pressure
		Uraemia
		Vestibular neuronitis

For references see [16].

Motor components of the vomiting reflex

While the often spectacular ejection of upper gastro-intestinal contents is the most obvious (and public) component of the vomiting reflex, it is in reality only the culmination of a series of motor events involving both the autonomic and somatic divisions of the nervous system. For convenience we will divide the reflex into two separate but usually consecutive phases: pre-ejection and ejection.

Pre-ejection phase

The pre-ejection or prodromal phase is characterized by the sensation of nausea, the physiological basis of which is poorly understood (see later). There are a number of visible signs such as cold sweating, cutaneous vasoconstriction and pupil dilation mediated by sympathetic nerves, and salivation mediated by parasympathetic nerves. In addition, changes in visceral function occur such as the onset of tachycardia and a reduction in gastric secretion, probably both mediated by sympathetic activation. Immediately prior to the onset of the ejection phase there is a profound relaxation of the proximal stomach mediated by vagal efferent nerves activating post-ganglionic neurons in the stomach wall. These neurons probably use vasoactive intestinal polypeptide as their neurotransmitter. In conjunction with this, a retrograde giant contraction (RGC) originates in the mid-small intestine and travels towards the stomach. The RGC is under vagal control and the transmitter involved is acetylcholine. These two gut motor events are of particular interest as they can be argued to have clear functions in the reflex, the gastric relaxation serving to confine orally ingested toxin to the stomach and the RGC returning any contaminated intestinal contents to the stomach ready for ejection [2]. The pre-ejection phase is usually, but not invariably, followed by the ejection phase.

Ejection phase

This phase comprises retching and vomiting with oral expulsion of gut contents only occurring during vomiting. The function of retching is unclear but it may be involved in overcoming the multi-component anti-reflux barrier present in the region of the gastro-oesophageal junction. Both retching and vomiting principally involve contractions of the somatic muscles of the abdomen (rectus abdominis and superior oblique) and diaphragm. During retching the abdominal muscles and the entire diaphragm contract synchronously whereas during vomiting the peri-oesophageal diaphragm relaxes — presumably to facilitate passage of gastric contents into the oesophagus and hence to the outside world [3]. The motor patterns and the resulting pressure changes are summarized in Fig. 2. Thus, the actual expulsion of gastric contents is due to compression of the stomach by the descending diaphragm and the contracting abdominal muscles under the influence of somatic motor neurons (see [4] for references). During retching and vomiting, all animals adopt a characteristic posture presumably to optimize compression of the stomach by the somatic muscles and to minimize strain on muscle groups and structures not involved in vomiting.

► Both nausea and vomiting are components of the body's defensive system against ingested poisons: vomiting is the physical act of ejecting poisons from the body while the nausea that usually accompanies it indicates to the animal that the contaminated food recently eaten should be avoided in future.
► In a clinical context most forms of vomiting do not lead to removal of the emetic stimulus (e.g. cytotoxic drug, anaesthetic), as it is present in the circulation and not in the gut lumen; however, the stimuli involved probably act via the same pathways and mechanisms that have evolved for the detection of orally ingested toxins in foods.
► The vomiting reflex can be divided into two phases: the pre-ejection phase involves relaxation of the proximal stomach in conjunction with an RGC in the small intestine; the ejection phase comprises oral expulsion of gastric contents brought about by compression of the stomach due to contraction of the diaphragm and the abdominal muscles.

Organization of the vomiting reflex

As we have seen above, the motor components of the reflex are mediated by both autonomic and somatic nerves. These motor pathways all

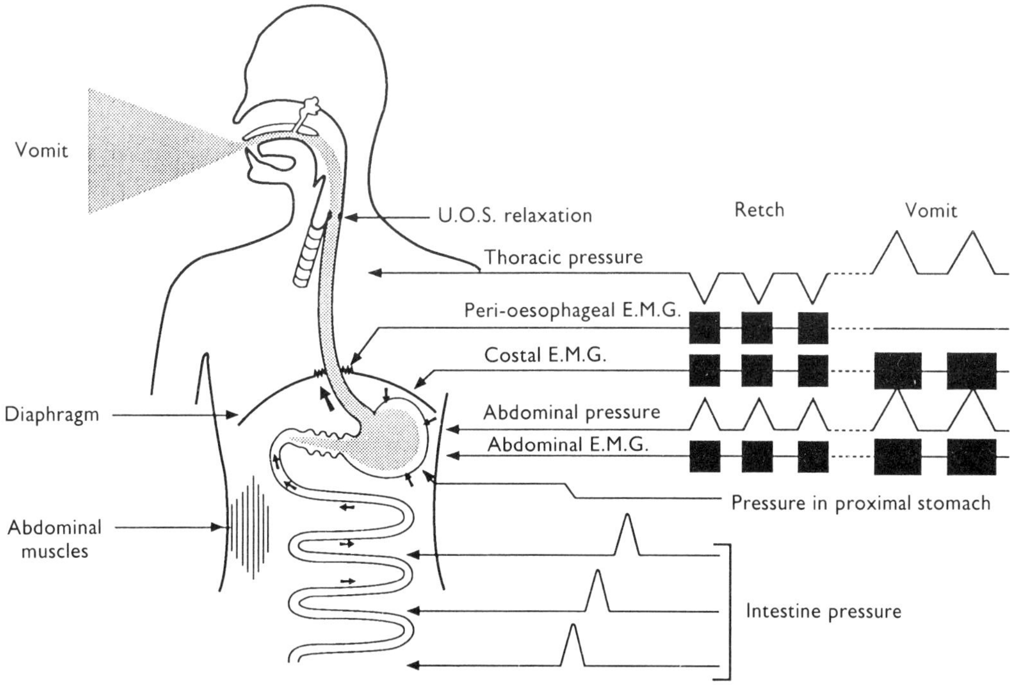

Fig. 2. A summary of the major gastro-intestinal and somatic motor changes that occur in association with retching and vomiting

Note that retching does not begin until the retrograde contraction in the intestine has reached the stomach and that the stomach relaxes prior to the initiation of this contraction. The main difference between retching and vomiting is in the motor activity of the two parts of the diaphragm. Abbreviations used: EMG, electromyogram; UOS, upper oesophageal sphincter. (Adapted from [4].)

have non-emetic functions. For example, the vagal non-adrenergic, non-cholinergic innervation of the stomach mediates gastric relaxation for the storage of food, and the phrenic nerve contracts the diaphragm for inspiration. In the vomiting reflex, these and many other motor pathways are activated in a unique pattern. Vomiting can be considered to be a stereotyped motor programme involving co-ordination between many physiological systems and between the autonomic and somatic components of the nervous system. An impression of the degree of co-ordination can be gained from the observation that the RGC in the small intestine is not initiated until the proximal stomach has relaxed and retching does not start until the RGC has reached the stomach [2].

The term 'vomiting centre' has been used widely to describe the central emetic co-ordinating mechanism. As in other areas of physiology, such terminology is now only used as a convenient shorthand for the co-ordinating system and as a substitute for a description of the neuro-anatomical substrate subserving such a function.

The co-ordination of the motor components of the vomiting reflex occurs in the brain stem (Fig. 3). It is here that the vagal motor neurons supplying the gut and heart originate in the dorsal motor vagal nucleus and nucleus ambiguous [5]. In addition, the dorsal and ventral respiratory groups regulating the phrenic nerve output from the cervical spinal cord are located in the brain stem, as are the pre-sympathetic neurons which maintain sympathetic tone to the heart and blood vessels. The output of these nuclei must be co-ordinated to produce the characteristic vomiting pattern described above. A promising candidate for this task is the nucleus tractus solitarius. This is probably the major integrative nucleus for visceral afferent information and, in addition, the ventral portion forms the dorsal respiratory neuronal group involved in

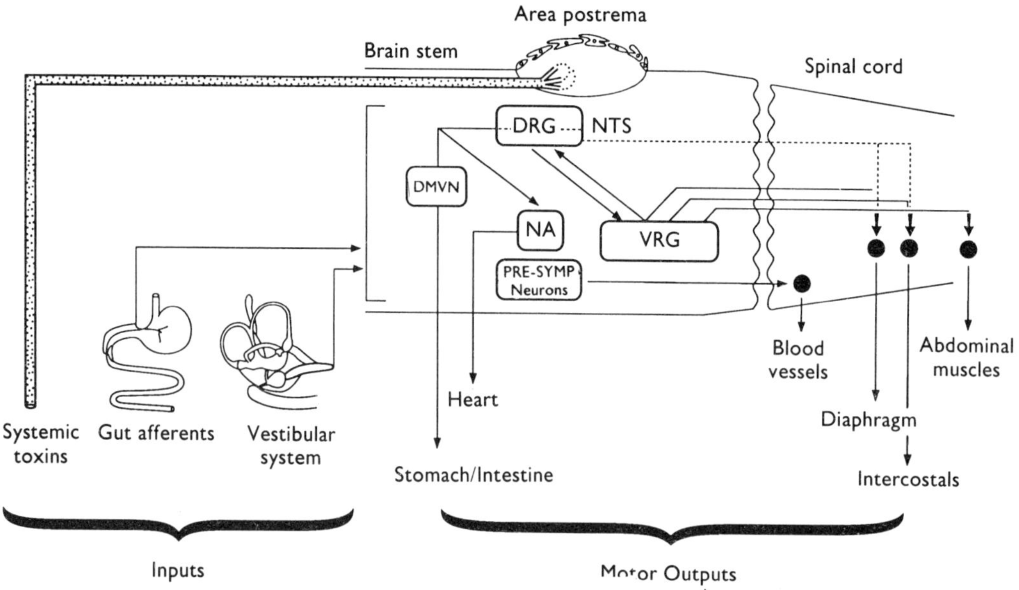

Fig. 3. Some of the brain stem nuclei involved in the visceral and somatic motor components of the vomiting reflex
Abbreviations used: DMVN, dorsal motor vagal nucleus; DRG, dorsal respiratory group of neurons; NA, nucleus ambiguous; NTS, nucleus tractus solitarius; PRE-SYMP neurons, pre-sympathetic group of neurons located in the ventrolateral medulla; VRG, ventral respiratory group of neurons. Adapted from [11].

the regulation of respiration [3]. Another candidate for the co-ordinating area is the parvicellular reticular formation and this has been reported to have many of the neuro-anatomical connections consistent with such a role [6]. When these central pathways receive the appropriate signal the entire visceral and somatic components constituting the vomiting reflex will be evoked. The mechanisms and pathways by which this activation occurs are described below.

Detection of emetic stimuli

Experiments in man and animals have identified abdominal vagal afferents and the area postrema as the systems involved in triggering many types of emesis. These will be discussed in detail below. Vomiting can also be activated from the vestibular apparatus and the cerebral cortex: a discussion of these pathways is beyond the scope of this chapter, although their role in induction of emesis in a clinical context is described later.

Abdominal vagal afferents

Afferent fibres contribute at least 80% of the fibres in the abdominal vagus and the majority of these are non-myelinated with conduction velocities of <2.5 m s^{-1}. They supply the entire tract from the oesophagus to the first part of the colon, although the upper gut appears to be most densely innervated [7]. The involvement of abdominal vagal afferents in emesis has been identified from studies in which the vomiting induced by stimuli such as hypertonic (1 M) sodium chloride in the stomach or gastric overdistension was abolished by abdominal vagotomy. In addition, electrical stimulation of abdominal vagal afferents readily induces emesis whereas splanchnic afferent stimulation is without effect (see [4, 8]).

The abdominal vagal afferents can be categorized into muscle afferents and mucosal afferents [9], and their properties in relation to their roles in emesis will be outlined briefly.

Muscle afferents

These afferents have receptive fields in the muscle layers of the gut wall and are thought to have their receptive elements located in series with the muscle. These properties are ideal for monitoring the degree of distension of various gut regions (particularly the proximal stomach with its food storage function) and the level of rhythmic contractile activity. Overdistension of the stomach, and notably the gastric antrum, can induce vomiting. This occurs by activation of these mechanoreceptive vagal afferents.

Mucosal afferents

These afferents have non-myelinated fibres and receptive fields in the mucosa. They are ideally located for monitoring various features of the luminal environment although their precise characteristics and functions are still a matter of some dispute. In general, they may be regarded as 'polymodal' with individual afferents responding to one or more of the following stimuli: stroking the mucosa, altered luminal osmolarity, acid, alkali, temperature or nutrients (glucose, amino acid, fatty acids). Their precise function in digestion is still unclear. This class of afferent can also be activated by hypertonic stimuli and by copper sulphate. Both these stimuli can induce emesis in man and animals within a few minutes after oral ingestion.

It is likely that these afferents are responsible for the identification of potential ingested poisons, although how this is achieved is still unclear [10].

Activation of the mucosal vagal afferents by toxins in the gut lumen is a potent stimulus for vomiting and, therefore, if a toxin present in the circulation can access the receptive region in the gut wall, emesis may result. Some of the mucosal afferents in the upper small intestine have terminals closely related to the 5-hydroxytryptamine (5-HT; serotonin)-containing enterochromaffin cells located in the mucosa. 5-HT can sensitize and evoke a discharge in abdominal vagal afferents. Hence, a toxin (systemic or luminal) could evoke emesis by inducing the release of 5-HT rather than by a direct effect on the nerve terminal [11]. This type of mechanism goes some way to explaining why such a diverse range of agents can induce emesis and why it is not necessary to postulate highly specialized detection systems. There are also similarities here to the airway vagal afferents which can induce cough (see Chapter 10).

Area postrema

The area postrema is a circumventricular organ (others include subcommissural organ, subfornical organ and the organum vasculosum of the lamina terminalis; [12]) located at the caudal extremity of the floor of the fourth ventricle. It is highly vascularized, receiving its blood supply from the anterior inferior cerebellar and spinal arteries. In common with other circumventricular organs it is 'outside' the blood–brain barrier mainly because the capillaries are fenestrated [13]. In addition, the cerebrospinal fluid–brain barrier is known to be incomplete, as quite large tracer molecules (e.g. horseradish peroxidase) in the cerebrospinal fluid can enter the area postrema. These features suggest a chemoreceptive function. The pioneering studies by Borison and Wang [14] showed that ablation of the area postrema abolished the response to a number of systemically administered emetic agents [e.g. morphine — an opiate receptor agonist, and apomorphine — a dopamine (D_2) receptor agonist]. These studies led to the proposal that the area postrema was the 'emetic chemoreceptor trigger zone' (CTZ). While there is little dispute that vomiting can be induced by activation of the area postrema via its known neuronal connections with the nucleus tractus solitarius (see Fig. 3), the use of the term 'emetic chemoreceptor trigger zone' has led to the widespread but incorrect assumption that emesis induced by *any* agent in the blood stream must be via this structure.

The involvement of the area postrema in emesis is most convincingly demonstrated using drugs acting on specific neurotransmitter receptors (e.g. morphine and apomorphine) rather than natural orally ingested toxins. Such studies may indicate that the area postrema is not the actual detector but only part of the pathway for emesis. If vomiting is considered in a biological context, where toxins are most likely to enter the body by ingestion, then it is strange that a detection system should be located at a post-absorptive site in the central nervous system. Triggering emesis from this site would not rid the body of the toxin that is already absorbed and which may already be damaging the tissues. The area postrema could be regarded as an additional, but final line of defence after the gut detection systems (Fig. 1).

The area postrema is reported to have a more general chemosensitive role and has been implicated to varying degrees in the regulation of food intake, sodium balance, respiration, arousal and blood pressure [15]. Thus, the emetic role may be more one aspect of this general chemosensitivity rather than a specific function. In the rat, which lacks a vomiting reflex, the area postrema is involved in the genesis of conditioned taste aversions.

A further problem with assessing the role of the area postrema is that the abdominal vagal afferents project to the portion of the nucleus tractus solitarius which lies just underneath the area postrema — the subnucleus gelatinosus or area sub-postrema. Thus, when the area postrema is lesioned it is quite likely that there is some damage to these vagal afferents and hence it would be possible to conclude (erroneously) that an emetic agent actually acting at the level of the gut was apparently acting on the area postrema (Fig. 4).

▶ Many types of emesis are triggered by the abdominal vagal afferents and the area postrema in the brain stem.
▶ Afferent fibres supply the entire gastro-intestinal tract from the oesophagus to the colon and consist of two types: mechanoreceptive afferents in the muscle signal the level of contraction and distension; mucosal afferents monitor the nature of the luminal contents and identify potential ingested toxins.
▶ The area postrema is a post-absorptive detection system in the brain stem which acts as a final line of defence against ingested poisons; its emetic role appears to be one aspect only of a more general chemoreceptor function.

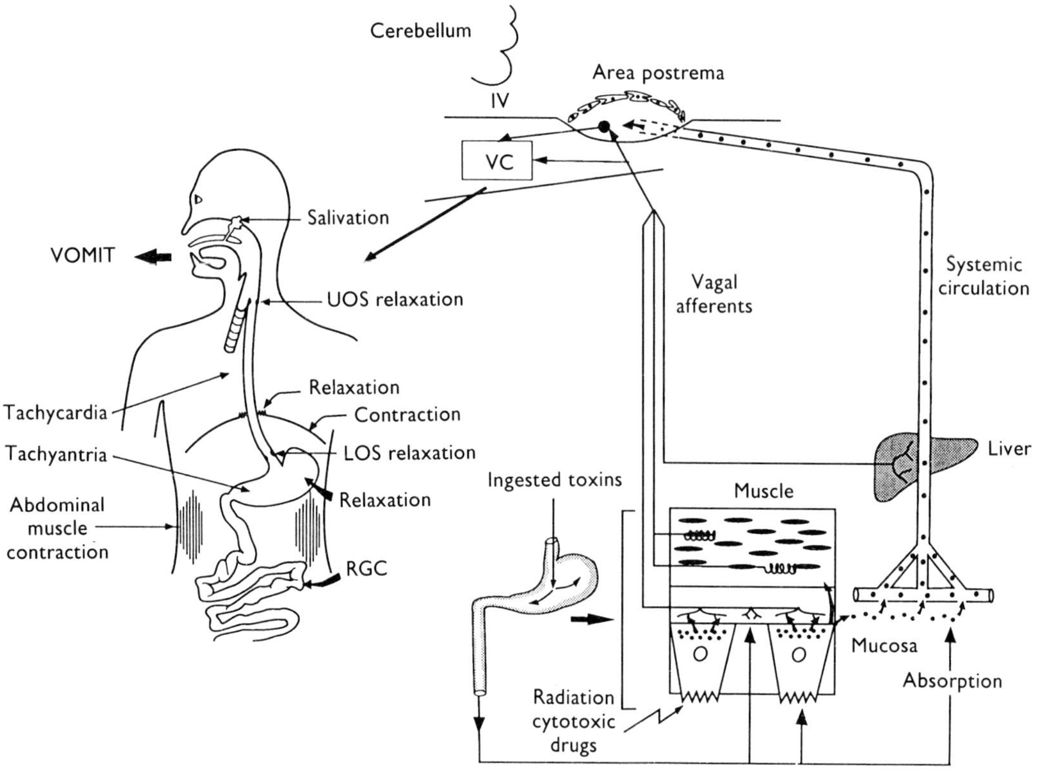

Fig. 4. A summary of the motor, afferent and central pathways of the somatic reflex
Abbreviations used: LOS, lower oesophageal sphincter; RGC, retrograde giant contraction; UOS, upper oesophageal sphincter; VC, vomiting centre; IV, fourth ventricle. See text for details. Adapted from [11].

The mechanism of vomiting induced by some clinical stimuli and the basis of anti-emetic action

As we discussed earlier, vomiting occurs in a very wide range of clinical conditions (Table 1) [16]. It is clearly impossible to review the mechanism by which each induces the emetic response and so a number of the more commonly encountered types have been selected to illustrate some of the mechanisms. For each stimulus the therapeutic approach and its rational basis is outlined briefly.

Gastro-intestinal motility disorders

Mechanism

Nausea, vomiting, early satiety, bloating and abdominal discomfort are often the first signs of disordered motility in the upper gastro-intestinal tract. Several types of motor disorder may be recognized, all of which lead to a delay in the movement of contents [17]. Two examples are given below.

(i) A delay or cessation (stasis) in gastric emptying may be brought about by impaired antral motility [18] or excessive relaxation of the gastric body. This may occur in patients with diabetic neuropathy in which there is damage to the vagal motor fibres and where a relationship is seen between the delay in gastric emptying and the incidence of vomiting. In diseases where there is damage to the myenteric plexus or the smooth muscle (e.g. systemic sclerosis) motility may be disordered. Emptying may also be delayed if the pattern of contractions in the antrum and duodenum is abnormal [19, 20]. It is not unusual for patients vomiting in the morning to bring up the meal eaten the previous evening, and in some cases the delay in gastric emptying may be so profound that food ingested several days earlier may be present in the vomit.

(ii) The movement of contents from the stomach to the duodenum will also be impaired if the pyloric sphincter between the two regions is in a spasm or if there is a mechanical obstruction in the lumen. This occurs in hypertrophic pyloric stenosis seen in neonates usually in the first two months of life [21].

Whatever causes delay in the movement of luminal contents the effect is the same: distension of the upper intestine or stomach. Experiments in animals have shown that vomiting can be induced by overdistension, particularly of gut regions such as the gastric antrum which have little storage capacity. In patients being treated for obesity using gastric balloons, nausea and vomiting are common side effects observed over the first 18 h after insertion [22]. Similarly, rapid distension of the stomach such as may occur in drinking a yard of ale in <20 s is an adequate stimulus for nausea and vomiting.

The main mechanism by which distension induces vomiting is most likely by intense activation of the abdominal vagal afferent mechanoreceptors (see above). However, following some surgical interventions to the gut, other mechanisms such as the release of endogenous chemicals from the gut could cause emesis. This must occur via an action on the area postrema since vomiting occurs in the presence of a vagotomy following procedures such as Roux-en-y anastomosis in which the vagus is cut, the proximal jejunum anastomosed to the gastric antrum, and the blind-ended duodenal segment side-anastomosed to the terminal jejunum.

Treatment

If the vomiting is due to mechanical obstruction, such as in hypertrophic pyloric stenosis, then surgery may be used successfully. If the problem is of a functional nature due to impaired motility, however, then drugs which stimulate gastric motility (e.g. cisapride, metoclopramide) and restore emptying to normal offer the best approach. It is important to realize that the vomiting mechanism itself is not being targeted by the drug but that the drug is being used to remove the stimulus of distension activating the pathway.

Food poisoning

Mechanism

Although we argued that the primary role of the vomiting reflex is to protect against accidental ingestion of toxins, the mechanism by which 'food poisoning' induces vomiting is very poorly understood.

Some toxins from plants and animals appear to induce emesis by virtue of their neuroactive properties which often involve opening the sodium channel. Examples of such toxins are veratridine (a plant alkaloid) or batrachotoxin (from the skin of a South American frog). Other ionic conductances are modified by the seafood toxins, brevetoxin and ciguatoxin, which come from dinoflagellate organisms found in some reef feeding fish in tropical areas [23]. These could induce emesis by activating gastro-intestinal vagal afferents as outlined earlier, or possibly by a direct action on the area postrema. The alkaloids (including emetine which is structurally related to the protein synthesis inhibitor cycloheximide) extracted from the root of the South American plant *Uragoga ipecacuanha* are used clinically in the form of syrup of ipecacuanha to induce vomiting in cases of drug overdose. Animal studies indicate that the mechanism is mainly via activation of vagal afferents with a central component if an appreciable quantity is absorbed.

A common organism responsible for food poisoning is the *Staphylococcus* bacterium producing enterotoxin B. Nausea, vomiting, abdominal cramping and diarrhoea typically occur within 1–4 h of ingestion [24]. Studies in the monkey demonstrated that the emetic response to oral toxin can be abolished either by area postrema ablation or abdominal denervation. These apparent contradictory observations can be reconciled if the toxin acts at the level of the gut and the emetic signal is relayed via the area postrema. Interestingly, injection of the toxin into the cerebro-spinal fluid failed to induce emesis, thus supporting the idea of the area postrema as a relay rather than a detector.

The way in which the toxin activates the afferents is not known but a mechanism involving the release of 5-HT from the enterochromaffin cell appears a likely possibility, especially as such a mechanism has been implicated in diarrhoea induced by *Escherichia coli* and *Vibrio cholerae* (see Chapters 3 and 7).

Acute episodes of non-bacterial gastroenteritis characterized by nausea, vomiting and diarrhoea are reported to be the commonest cause of gut symptoms in North America. Rota and Norwalk viruses are often implicated as causative agents but little is known of how such agents induce these symptoms [25].

Treatment

In general it is clearly not desirable to block vomiting induced by food poisoning any more than blocking diarrhoea, since both serve to remove the toxin from the body. Treatment usually consists of metabolic support until the vomiting subsides after a few days.

Anti-cancer chemotherapy and radiotherapy

Mechanism

The vomiting induced by some anti-cancer therapies provides a good example of nausea and vomiting induced as a 'side effect' of therapy, which may have serious implications for the patient. The cytotoxic drugs used in the treatment of tumours induce nausea and vomiting to varying degrees. For example, the vinca alkaloids and 5-fluoro-uracil produce these symptoms in $<30\%$ of patients, while cisplatin affects $>90\%$ [26]. With the latter agent, nausea and vomiting begin within a few hours of administration and continue in the majority of patients for 24 h and in some for several days (called delayed emesis). This may occur with each cycle of vomiting and there are reports of patients who decline further courses of potentially curative therapy because the vomiting and continual nausea is unbearable. Radiotherapy, also used for treatment of tumours, induces nausea and vomiting but this can be reduced considerably by using local radiation as opposed to whole-body radiation and by fractionating the dose. However, radiation emesis is still a problem in patients requiring large whole-body doses of radiation to suppress the bone marrow prior to transplantation, and in those accidentally exposed to high doses of radiation such as occurred at Chernobyl.

In the past 5 years our knowledge of the way in which radiation and cytotoxic drugs induce emesis has changed dramatically mainly because of basic scientific studies in the ferret. Experiments revealed that the emetic response to whole-body radiation and to the systemically administered cytotoxic drugs, such as cisplatin and cyclophosphamide, was abolished or markedly reduced by abdominal vagotomy [8]. Previous studies in other species (cat) and subsequent studies in the ferret have shown that area postrema ablation can also have a similar effect (see [11]). These and other experiments suggested that such stimuli induced emesis primarily by activation of abdominal vagal afferents via a pathway involving the area postrema or an intimately related region (Fig. 4). Interestingly, the upper abdomen is the most sensitive site for radiation induction of emesis [27].

The vomiting induced by these stimuli is of particular interest because, in contrast to vomiting elicited by gastric distension and ingested toxins, the act of vomiting is not directed towards removing the emetic stimulus and therefore may be considered to be inappropriate. However, as far as the animal is concerned, the mechanism which is there to detect ingested toxins is being activated and hence the correct response is elicited even though the response is ineffective.

Treatment

Clinical studies in the early 1980s revealed that vomiting induced by anti-cancer therapies could be reduced using 'high' doses of metaclopramide. Studies by Miner and Sanger [28] at Beecham Pharmaceuticals and Costall, Domeney, Naylor and Tattersall [29] at the University of Bradford showed that the anti-emetic effect of metoclopramide was not due to its dopamine (D2) receptor antagonist actions or its gut motility stimulant action mediated by the release of acetylcholine. Instead, they revealed the effect to be caused by another pharmacological action of metoclopramide, that of antagonism of the 5-HT sub-type 3 receptor (5-HT_3). More selective and potent 5-HT_3 receptor antagonists were synthesized by both Beecham and Glaxo and these compounds (Kytril and Zofran) have been shown to be extremely effective in the clinic, specifically for the treatment of radiation and cytotoxic-induced nausea and vomiting [30, 31].

The site at which these drugs act is still under investigation but it has been proposed that their main effect is to block the activation of abdominal vagal afferents by 5-HT released from the enterochromaffin cells in the gut that is stimulated by radiation and cytotoxic drugs [11]. This does not exclude an additional central site(s), probably in the brain stem.

Motion sickness

Mechanism

Nausea and vomiting can be induced by travel in car, aeroplane, ship, spacecraft and even on camels [32, 33]. The word 'nausea' derived from the Greek for ship attests to the long known link between certain forms of motion and sickness.

Motion sickness differs from the other stimuli we have considered in that there is no hard evidence for an involvement of the area postrema or the gastro-intestinal afferents. The key element in the genesis of most forms of motion sickness is stimulation of the vestibular system. The visual system is not essential except in the case of illusory self motion such as occurs in IMAX cinemas or fixed aircraft simulators. The visual system plays some role in inducing emesis when there is a mismatch or sensory conflict between the visual and vestibular systems such that information from one sensory system is unsupported or contradicted by that from another. The signals from the vestibular apparatus pass to the vestibular nuclei by primary vestibular fibres in cranial nerve VIII and then to the vestibular cerebellum. The output from the vestibular cerebellum projects to the brain stem structures involved in generating the visceral and somatic components of the vomiting reflex. Removal of the cerebellar nodulus in dogs prevents motion sickness. Opportunities for interactions between the visual and vestibular system exist in the cerebellum and vestibular nuclei [34].

Motion sickness itself is not really a clinical problem, but, in Meniere's disease, labyrinthitis and vestibular neuronitis, abnormal discharge from the vestibular nerve results in vertigo and hence nausea and vomiting. Vertigo may also result if the hair cells in the vestibular labyrinths are damaged by ototoxic drugs. In evolutionary terms motion sickness is one of the hardest forms of vomiting to rationalize as the vomiting does not lead to removal of the stimulus.

A variety of animals, including fish, vomit in response to motion. Even animals such as the rat which do not vomit appear to experience malaise. It is even possible to induce a taste aversion by pairing the taste stimulus with motion. One attractive hypothesis which helps to explain motion sickness was proposed by Treisman [35]. He suggested that motion sickness was in fact a component of the defence system against ingested toxins. This was based on the observation that poisoned animals are likely to become unsteady and hence there will be stimulation of the vestibular system and probably vestibular–visual mismatch leading to initiation of vomiting.

Treatment

In travel sickness the probability of inducing emesis can be reduced if the subject has a clear view of the horizon and occupies a position in the vehicle where vertical motion is at a minimum. On a ship the best place would be on deck so that the horizon is visible to give a clear and stable frame of reference and amidships where vertical motion is reduced. Repeated exposure to motion stimuli leads to natural adaptation, but, in those undergoing aircrew training who may be slow to adapt, this may be augmented by desensitization treatment using laboratory-based stimuli [34].

The most widespread pharmacological treatments for motion sickness are antagonism of central muscarinic cholinergic receptors by hyoscine or scopolamine and blockade of central histamine (H1) receptors by cinnarizine or promethazine. For labyrinthine disorders and vertigo, cholinergic receptor antagonists are also used but a common treatment is prochlorperazine. This drug has a complex pharmacological action with antagonist activity at dopamine receptors (D1 and D2), histamine receptors (H1), adrenergic receptors ($\alpha 1$) and cholinergic receptors. The clinical action is generally ascribed to its actions on dopamine and histamine receptors.

Pregnancy

Mechanisms

Two very distinct types of vomiting may occur during pregnancy and these will be discussed separately.

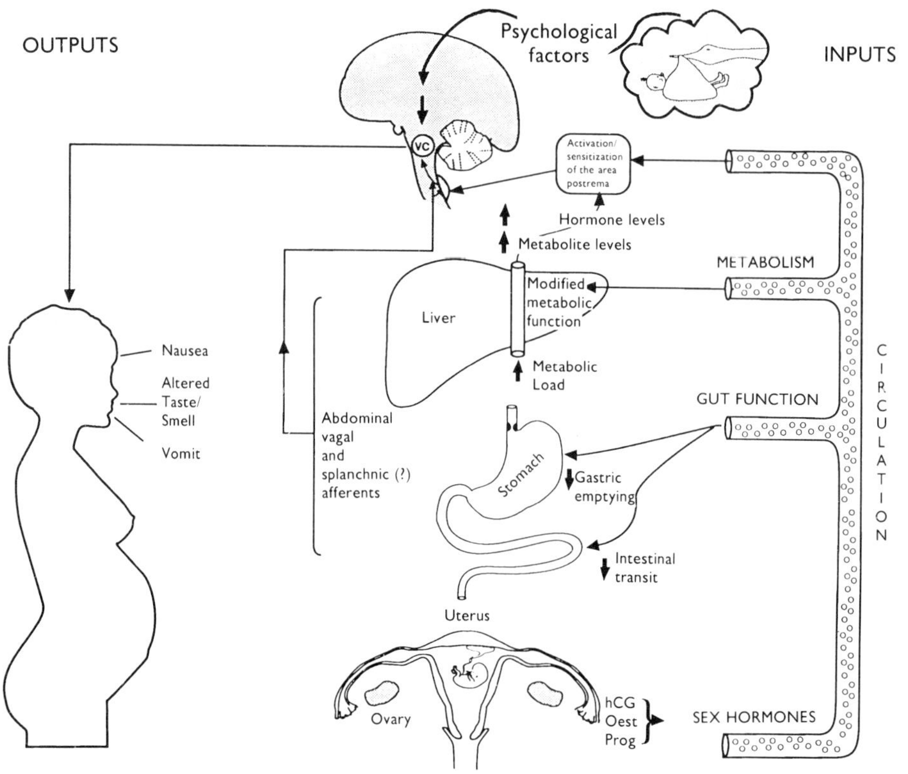

Fig. 5. A summary of some of the mechanisms that may be involved in pregnancy sickness

Abbreviations used: hCG, human chorionic gonadotrophin; Oest, oestrogen; Prog, progesterone. Adapted from [36a].

(i) Pregnancy sickness is the typical nausea and vomiting associated with pregnancy, which is often called incorrectly 'morning sickness' although vomiting occurs at other times of the day as well. A recent suvey of 1000 pregnant women at St George's Hospital, London [36] revealed that some 80% had this form of sickness. Typically, nausea and vomiting begin within a few weeks of conception and may be the first indication of pregnancy for some women. The symptoms last throughout the first trimester. The possible mechanisms have been reviewed [36], but no single factor (except pregnancy!) has been identified (Fig. 5). The time course of the phenomenon does not correlate with the changing pattern of secretion of any of the sex hormones, with the possible exception of chorionic gonadotrophin (hCG). Even if we cannot understand the mechanism, can we rationalize the linkage of the biological function crucial for the survival of the species (i.e. pregnancy) with such highly aversive stimuli as nausea and vomiting of several months duration? During early pregnancy the foetus must be protected against maternal ingestion of abortifacient and teratogenic substances. The development of taste aversions, changes in perception of some tastes and the reduced threshold for nausea may be argued as limiting the range of foods consumed in pregnancy. Thus, the animal is less likely to consume novel and potentially toxic substances. This may give it a selective advantage. In rats the area postrema has been implicated in taste aversions, food palatability and nausea, and hence such changes may reflect a modification of area postrema function by unknown factors operating in pregnancy. The vomiting may therefore be an undesirable component of an otherwise advantageous adaptation to pregnancy.

(ii) Hyperemesis gravidarum is a rare form of vomiting, occurring in about one out of 1000 pregnancies. It is intractable, begins before the 20th week of pregnancy and leads to disturbed maternal nutrition and electrolyte balance which may require hospitalization. Coincidental conditions such as appendicitis and pre-eclampsia must be excluded. The basis of this sickness is unknown, although endocrine (particularly hCG), metabolic (impaired liver function) and even psychosomatic (attempt to eject the foetus) factors have all been implicated. Whatever the mechanism, the seriousness of the condition should not be underestimated as the electrolyte disturbances, which include hypokalaemia, may give rise to neurological and cardiac disturbances. The dramatic reduction in maternal deaths ascribed to hyperemesis, from 159 per million births in the 1930s in England and Wales to 3 per million in the 1950s is attributed to recognition of the significance of electrolyte imbalance. Interestingly, hyperemesis gravidarum has no effect on infant birth weight [37].

Treatment

Drug treatment for pregnancy ('morning') sickness is inappropriate for several reasons. First, there is an ever-present danger of foetal damage by any active agent. Second, the vomiting resolves itself after a few months. Third, as the mechanism behind the sickness is not known, it is difficult to identify a rational therapy targeted at a specific site. The drug Debendox [dicyclamine, doxylamine and pyridoxine (vitamin B6)] alleged to be responsible for foetal malformations was given to women for pregnancy sickness but this usage was not based on studies of the pharmacology of pregnancy sickness itself. Because animals appear not to suffer from vomiting in pregnancy, it is not possible to screen for such drugs in animal models.

The most beneficial action a doctor can take is to reassure the mother that 'morning' sickness is a normal response to pregnancy and that the foetus will not be harmed as a result. Some women find that changing the pattern of eating to frequent small meals helps Acupuncture and relaxation techniques have also been found to be beneficial in coping with pregnancy sickness.

> ▶ Gastro-intestinal motility disorders include impaired movement of luminal contents (stasis) and mechanical obstruction in the lumen; both problems result in distension of the upper intestine or stomach, thus activating the vomiting reflex.
>
> ▶ Toxins from ingested food are thought to be detected in the gut (possibly by a mechanism involving the local release of 5-HT), and the emetic signal relayed via vagal afferents to the brain stem.

▶ The pathways by which anti-cancer chemotherapy and radiotherapy induce emesis are thought to be similar to those involved in food poisoning: the stimuli act primarily at the abdominal vagal afferents via a pathway thought to involve the area postrema as a relay.
▶ Motion sickness is brought about by stimulation of the vestibular and (to a lesser extent) visual systems: vestibular–visual mismatch is the most likely cause of emesis.
▶ The function of pregnancy ('morning') sickness is thought to be to limit the range of food consumed in pregnancy, thus reducing the risk of toxin ingestion at the time when the foetus is most sensitive to teratogens.

Consequences of vomiting

While isolated episodes of vomiting may be only a minor inconvenience to an otherwise healthy individual, the consequences of protracted vomiting and nausea may be considerable (Fig. 6) and in some cases life-threatening. Some of these are outlined below and serve to illustrate the clinical significance of the search for anti-emetic therapies.

Physical

Vomiting is a physically demanding act which may place considerable stresses upon some body regions. There are reports of ribs breaking during violent vomiting. Protracted vomiting can lead to soreness of the abdominal muscles due to the frequent and intense activation which occurs rarely in other activities. Such activity would, of course, be painful and compromise wound healing if it occurred in the post-operative state following abdominal or pelvic surgery. The motor component of vomiting involves the cranial movement of the stomach and the rapid delivery of gastric contents into the oesophagus. These events may lead to herniation of the stomach into the thorax and tearing of the gastro-oesophageal mucosa with resultant haemorrhage (Mallory–Weiss syndrome) or even rupture of the oesophagus (Boerhave syndrome).

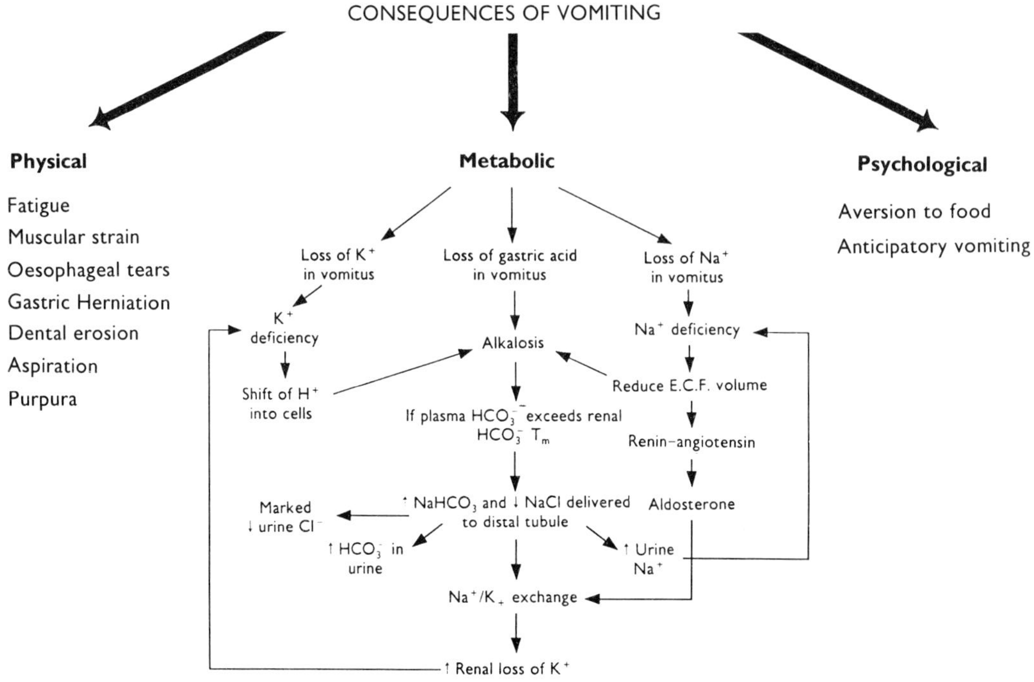

Fig. 6. The consequences of vomiting
Abbreviations used: ECF, extracellular fluid compartment; T_m, renal tubular maximum transport capacity. Modified from [11, 44].

The gastric contents are always acidic and their delivery into the mouth may lead to dental erosion. This is particularly noticeable in bulaemic patients who gorge and then make themselves vomit. It has been suggested that the salivation which precedes vomiting is an attempt to buffer the acidic vomit and hence protect the buccal cavity.

Aspiration of vomit or regurgitated food is a particular problem in unconscious or heavily sedated patients (e.g. immediately after surgery or in a coma) or in neonates with a weak lower oesophageal sphincter [21]. Aspiration may cause asphyxia, epithelial damage and aspiration pneumonia (a chemical pneumonitis) due to acid against which the airways have little defence.

Metabolic

Vomiting has two main metabolic consequences. Firstly, it leads to the expulsion of food and hence a degree of malnutrition, particularly in children. The accompanying sensation of nausea will blunt the desire for food. Secondly, the loss of gastric secretions leads to dehydration, and loss of hydrogen, sodium, potassium and chloride ions. The reduced plasma volume causes decreased renal perfusion and aldosterone secretion. The latter exacerbates the hypokalaemia (flow plasma $[K^+]$) and alkalosis. The loss of chloride ions and plasma increases renal bicarbonate ion reabsorption which contributes to the alkalosis and hypokalaemia. Hypophosphataemia may also occur. The ionic losses may be fatal because of the effects that they have on the function of excitable tissues such as cardiac and skeletal muscle and neurons.

Psychological

The psychological effects of protracted vomiting and nausea should not be underestimated in their importance as they may continue long after the vomiting itself has stopped. The main clinical problem is the development of 'anticipatory nausea and vomiting'. Patients receiving some chemotherapeutic agents (e.g. cisplatin) or large doses of radiation for the treatment of tumours may have prolonged (days) episodes of nausea and vomiting on each occasion that the therapy is given. The therapy becomes clearly associated with the side effect. Because of this association, in some patients the thought of therapy, the sight of the hospital or even, in one case, the oncologist may all trigger nausea and vomiting. The aversion to therapy may be so severe that further therapy is declined with potentially fatal results. In addition to the anticipatory response, patients may also develop taste aversions for foods which are eaten around the time of chemotherapy [38].

What is the physiological basis of nausea?

This chapter has reviewed the mechanisms by which the vomiting reflex can be triggered by a wide range of stimuli and described the motor components of the reflex. In general, the mechanisms account for most of the experimental and clinical observations and provide a framework within which the site of action of anti-emetic drugs can be considered. There are some fascinating outstanding problems such as the mechanism and function (if any) of pregnancy sickness and identification of the mechanisms by which a single dose of a chemotherapeutic agent such as cisplatin can induce vomiting for several days.

One of the major gaps in our knowledge is the mechanisms involved in the genesis of the sensation of nausea. Nausea has a clear biological function and is induced by all the stimuli which induce vomiting. In contrast to vomiting, which is a reflex motor response, nausea is a conscious sensation with associated changes in behaviour. There are certainly pathways by which information from vagal afferents and the area postrema could reach the visceral portion of the sensory cortex in the granular portion of the insular region [39], but whether such pathways could account for induction of nausea by psychological and motion stimuli is not clear.

Recent studies in man have identified two parameters which alter during nausea. Firstly, the frequency of electrical activity of the stomach muscle increases (tachygastria) and develops a dysrhythmic pattern. Secondly, there is a large (250 × in one study) rise in plasma vasopressin (ADH) but not oxytocin. This has been seen in response to apomorphine, illusory self motion and chemotherapeutic agents [40–43]. Whether these changes are involved in generating the sensation or whether they are a consequence has not yet been resolved.

I wish to thank Dr S. A. Whitehead for critical comments on the manuscript.

References

1. Pelchat, M. L. and Rozin, P. (1982) The special role of nausea in the acquisition of food dislikes by humans. Appetite **3**, 341–351
2. Lang, I. M. (1990) Digestive tract motor correlates of vomiting and nausea. Can. J. Physiol. Pharmacol. **68**, 242–253
3. Miller, A. D. (1990) Respiratory mechanics of vomiting. Can. J. Physiol. Pharmacol. **68**, 237–241
4. Andrews, P. L. R. and Hawthorn, J. (1988) The neurophysiology of vomiting. Clin. Gastroenterol. **2**, 141–168
5. Loewy, A. D. and Spyer, K. M. (1990) Vagal preganglionic neurons. In Central Regulation of Autonomic Functions (Loewy, A. D. and Spyer, K. M., eds.), pp. 68–87, Oxford University Press, Oxford
6. Mehler, W. R. (1983) Observations on the connectivity of the parvicellular reticular formation with respect to a vomiting centre. Brain Behav. Evol. **23**, 63–80
7. Andrews, P. L. R. (1986) Vagal afferent innervation of the gastro-intestinal tract. Progr. Brain Res. **67**, 65–86
8. Andrews, P. L. R., Davis, C. J., Bingham, S., Davidson, H. I. M., Hawthorn, J. and Maskell, L. (1990) The abdominal visceral innervation and the emetic reflex: Pathways pharmacology and plasticity. Can. J. Physiol. Pharmacol. **68**, 325–345
9. Grundy, D. G. and Scratcherd, T. (1989) Sensory afferents from the gastrointestinal tract. In Handbook of Physiology, Section 6, Vol. 1, part 1 (Wood, J. D., ed.), pp. 593–620, American Physiological Society, Bethesda, Maryland, U.S.A.
10. Grundy, D. G., Andrews, P. L. R. and Blackshaw, L. A. (1991) Neural correlates of the gastrointestinal motor changes in emesis. In Brain Gut Interactions (Tache, Y. and Wingate, D., eds.), pp. 325–338, CRC Press, Boca Raton, U.S.A.
11. Andrews, P. L. R. and Davis, C. J. (1993) The mechanism of emesis induced by anti-cancer therapies. In Emesis in Anti-cancer Therapy: Mechanisms and Treatment (Andrews, P. L. R. and Sanger, G. J., eds.), pp. 113–161, Chapman and Hall Medical, London
12. Landas, S., Fischer, J., Wilkin, L. D., Mitchell, L. D., Johnson, A. K., Turner, J. W., Theriac, M. and Moore, K. C. (1985) Demonstration of regional blood brain barrier permeability in human brain. Neurosci. Lett. **57**, 251–256
13. Leslie, R. A. (1986) Comparative aspects of the area postrema: fine structural considerations help to determine its function. Cell. Mol. Neurobiol. **6**, 95–120
14. Borison, H. L. and Wang, S. C. (1953) Physiology and pharmacology of vomiting. Pharmacol. Rev. **5**, 193–230
15. Borison, H. L. (1989) Area postrema: chemoreceptor circumventricular organ of the medulla oblongata. Progr. Neurobiol. **32**, 351–390
16. Davis, C. J., Lake-Bakaar, G. V. and Grahame-Smith, D. G. (1986) Nausea and Vomiting: Mechanisms and Treatment (Davis, C. J., Lake-Bakaar, G. V. and Grahame-Smith, D. G., eds.), p. 184, Springer-Verlag, Berlin, Heidelberg
17. Kumar, D. and Gustavsson, S. (1988) An Illustrated Guide to Gastrointestinal Motility, p. 470, John Wiley and Sons, Chichester
18. Kerlin, P. (1989) Postprandial antral hypomotility in patients with idiopathic nausea and vomiting. Gut **30**, 54–59
19. Geldof, H., Van der Schee, E. J., Van Blankenstein, M. and Grashuis, J. L. (1986) Electrogastrographic study of myoelectrical activity in patients with unexplained nausea and vomiting. Gut **27**, 799–808
20. Malagelada, J. R. and Stanghellini, V. (1985) Manometric evaluation of upper gut symptoms. Gastroenterology **88**, 1223–1231
21. Milla, P. J. (1988) Disorders of Gastrointestinal Motility in Childhood, p. 143, John Wiley and Sons, Chichester
22. Durrans, D. and Taylor, T. V. (1989) Comparison of weight loss with short term dietary and intragastric balloon treatment. Gut **30**, 565–568
23. Harris, J. B. (1986) Natural Toxins, Animal, Plant and Microbial, p. 353, Clarendon Press, Oxford
24. Elwell, M. R., Liu, C. T., Spertzel, R. O. and Beisel, W. R. (1975) Mechanism of oral enterotoxin B-induced emesis in the monkey. Proc. Soc. Exp. Biol. Med. **148**, 424–427
25. Meeroff, J. C., Schreiber, D. S., Trier, J. S. and Blacklow, N. R. (1980) Abnormal gastric motor function in viral gastroenteritis. Ann. Intern. Med. **92**, 370–373
26. Harris, A. L. and Cantwell, B. M. J. (1986) Mechanisms and treatment of cytotoxic induced nausea and vomiting. In Nausea and Vomiting: Mechanisms and Treatment (Davis, C. J., Lake-Bakaar, G. V. and Grahame-Smith, D. G., eds.), pp. 78–93, Springer-Verlag, Berlin, Heidelberg
27. Young, R. W. (1986) Mechanism and treatment of radiation induced nausea and vomiting. In Nausea and Vomiting: Mechanisms and Treatment (Davis, C. J., Lake-Bakaar, G. V. and Grahame-Smith, D. G., eds.), pp. 94–109, Springer-Verlag, Berlin, Heidelberg
28. Miner, W. and Sanger, G. J. (1986) Inhibition of cis-platinum induced vomiting by selective 5-hydroxytryptamine-M-receptor antagonism. Br. J. Pharmacol. **88**, 497–499
29. Costall, B., Domeney, A. M., Naylor, R. J. and Tattersall, F. D. (1986) 5-Hydroxytryptamine M-receptor antagonism to prevent cisplatin induced emesis. Neuropharmacology **25**, 957–961
30. Cassidy, J., Raina, V., Lewis, C., Adams, L., Soukop, M., Rapeport, W. G., Zussman, B. D., Rankin, E. M. and Kaye, S. B. (1988) Pharmacokinetics and anti-emetic efficacy of BRL 43694, a new selective 5HT-3 antagonist. Br. J. Cancer **58**, 651–653
31. Cubeddu, L. X., Hoffmann, I. S., Fuenmayor, N. T. and Finn, A. L. (1990) Efficacy of ondansetron and the role of serotonin in cisplatin-induced nausea and vomiting. New Engl. J. Med. **322**, 810–816
32. Reason, J. T. and Brand, J. J. (1975) Motion Sickness, p. 310, Academic Press, London
33. Crampton, G. H. (1990) Motion and Space Sickness, p. 451, CRC Press, Florida, U.S.A.
34. Stott, J. R. R. (1986) Mechanisms and treatment of motion illness. In Nausea and Vomiting: Mechanisms and Treatment (Davis, C. J., Lake-Bakaar, G. V. and Grahame-Smith, D. G., eds.), pp. 110–129, Springer-Verlag, Berlin, Heidelberg
35. Treisman, M. (1977) Motion sickness: an evolutionary hypothesis. Science **197**, 493–495
36. Whitehead, S. A., Andrews, P. L. R. and Chamberlain, G. V. P. (1992) Characterisation of nausea and vomiting in early pregnancy: a survey of 1000 women. J. Obstet. Gynaecol. **12**, 364–369

36a. Andrews, P. L. R. and Whitehead, S. A. (1990) Pregnancy sickness. News Physiol. Sci. **5**, 5–10

37. Fairweather, D. V. I. (1986) Mechanisms and treatment of nausea and vomiting in pregnancy. In Nausea and Vomiting: Mechanisms and Treatment (Davis, C. J., Lake-Bakaar, G. V. and Grahame-Smith, D. G., eds.), pp. 151–159, Springer-Verlag, Berlin, Heidelberg
38. Bernstein, I. L. (1978) Learned taste aversions in children receiving chemotherapy. Science **200**, 1302–1303
39. Cechetto, D. F. and Saper, C. B. (1990) Role of the cerebral cortex in autonomic function. In Central Regulation of Autonomic Functions (Loewy, A. D. and Spyer, K. M., eds.), pp. 308–323, Oxford University Press, Oxford
40. Nussey, S., Hawthorn, J., Page, S. R., Ang, V. T. Y. and Jenkins, J. S. (1988) Responses of plasma oxytocin and arginine vasopressin to nausea induced by apomorphine and ipecacuanha. Clin. Endocrinol. **28**, 297–304
41. Feldman, M., Samson, W. K. and O'Dorisio, T. M. (1988) Apomorphine-induced nausea in humans: release of vaso-

pressin and pancreatic polypeptide. Gastroenterology **95**, 721–726

42. Koch, K. L., Summy-Long, J., Bingaman S., Sperry, N. and Stern, R. M. (1990) Vasopressin and oxytocin response to illusory self-motion and nausea in man. J. Clin. Endocrinol. Metab. **71**, 1269–1275
43. Fisher, R. D., Rentschler, R. E., Nelson, J. C., Godfrey, T. E. and Wilbur, D. W. (1982) Elevation of plasma ADH associated with chemotherapy induced emesis in man. Cancer Treat. Rep. **66**, 25–29
44. Feldman, M. (1989) Vomiting. In Gastrointestinal Disease (Sleisenger, M. H. and Fordtran, J. S., eds.), pp. 222–238, W. B Saunders and Co, Philadelphia, U.S.A.

Achalasia
A disorder of the oesophagus in which there is a defect of normal peristalsis in the lower two thirds (smooth muscle portion) of the oesophagus and an elevated tone (tightening) of the lower oesophageal sphincter. Thus, the passage of food from the mouth to the stomach is impeded.

Adrenergic
A neuron using noradrenaline or, in rare cases, adrenaline as a neurotransmitter. Application of noradrenaline to the target tissue innervated should mimic (at least in part) the response to nerve stimulation. The term 'adrenergic' has often been used synonymously with 'sympathetic', but such usage should be avoided in view of the demonstration of non-adrenergic components of neurotransmission in the sympathetic division of the nervous system.

Anaphylaxis
A condition of hypersensitivity to certain antigens, that can be induced experimentally, for example by the injection of a 'sensitizing' dose that renders an animal hypersusceptible to a subsequent 'assault' dose. The anaphylactic response is probably the result of an antigen–antibody reaction occurring in tissue cells that have removed the antibody from the blood and fixed it to themselves. Substances producing anaphylaxis in humans include horse serum and bacterial antigens. Histamine injected intravenously can mimic an anaphylactic response.

Apnoea
The cessation of breathing (leading to asphyxia) or a temporary pause in breathing after forced respiration.

Apomorphine
*An artificial alkaloid prepared by the removal of water from the molecule of morphine; it stimulates the CTZ (*see *Area postrema) and is therefore used as an emetic in acute poisoning. In spite of its name it is a dopamine D_2 receptor agonist and not an opiate receptor agonist.*

Area postrema
A circumventricular organ located in the caudal extremity of the fourth ventricle. It is outside the blood-brain and blood-cerebrospinal fluid barriers. Although it has been implicated in emesis and is often called the 'chemoreceptor trigger zone for emesis' (CTZ), this is only one aspect of a more generalized chemoreceptor role.

ASL
Airway-surface liquid covering the airway epithelial surface: it consists of a surface gel derived from goblet cells and mucus glands, on top of a sol layer, and it is propelled by cilia; important as a protective barrier and for swallowing and expectoration.

ATP
Adenosine-5'-triphosphate — proposed to be one of the purigenic neurotransmitters implicated in non-adrenergic, non-cholinergic transmission and modulation, the other being adenosine.

Atropine
A poisonous alkaloid found in solanceous plants, in particular, Atropa belladonna. *It blocks (antagonizes) the effects of acetylcholine (acting on muscarinic cholinergic receptors) on structures in effector organs supplied by post-ganglionic cholinergic nerves; e.g. it diminishes secretion in gastric, bronchial and salivary glands, and relaxes airway smooth muscle. Its uses include the relief of asthma and the diminution of secretions before general anaesthesia.*

Autacoid
A term derived from the Greek 'autos' (self) and 'akos' (medicinal agent or remedy). It is a rather imprecise term used to describe a number of substances that are produced by the body, usually having a brief duration of action locally near the site of synthesis. Autocoids are often called 'local hormones' as, although they have hormone-like actions, they do not enter the circulation. Examples of autocoids include 5-hydroxy-tryptamine, histamine, bradykinin and eicosanoids.

Bradycardia
Slowing of the heart rate caused by, for example, activation of vagal efferent fibres supplying the sino-atrial node (pacemaker) tissue.

C-fibre
A non-myelinated nerve with a conduction velocity less than 2.5 m s^{-1}. Many sensory (afferent) C-fibres can be discharged by acute application of capsaicin to their terminal receptor region.

Capsaicin
One of the pungent extracts from red peppers of the genus Capsicum *used experimentally to investigate the function of peripheral afferent C-fibres. Chemically, it is a vanillyl amide derivative: 8-methyl-*N*-vanillyl-6-nonenamide. When given systemically to animals in the first few days of life, it causes selective destruction of a large population of afferent C-fibres, such that the effect of their destruction can be studied when the animals reach maturity. In the adult animal, it causes initial activation of afferent C-fibres followed by desensitization, and with chronic administration irreversible damage may result.*

CF
Cystic fibrosis — a disorder of the mucus-secreting glands of the lungs, pancreas, mouth and gastro-intestinal tract, as well as of the sweat glands of the skin. In this condition, recurrent endobronchial infections cause progressive destruction of the lung tissue, while pancreatic exocrine failure leads to malabsorption of nutrients, chronic diarrhoea and weight loss. It is the most common inherited genetic disorder in caucasian children and is caused by a defect in a single gene on chromosome 7, which affects the transport of ions and water across epithelial cell membranes.

CFTR
Cystic fibrosis transmembrane conductance regulator — the protein encoded by the cystic fibrosis gene. With several sequences that are similar to those found in transmembrane proteins, it is thought to be involved in regulating the opening of chloride channels.

ChAT
Choline-acetyltransferase — catalyses the synthesis of acetylcholine from acetyl CoA and choline.

Cholinergic
A neuron using acetylcholine as a neurotransmitter. Application of acetylcholine to the target tissue innervated should mimic (at least in part) the response to nerve stimulation. The term 'cholinergic' has often been used synonomously with 'parasympathetic', but such usage should be avoided in view of the demonstration of non-cholinergic components of neurotransmission in the parasympathetic division of the nervous system.

Cisplatin
A co-ordination complex of the metal platinum, used as a cytotoxic drug in the treatment of solid tumours (e.g. testicular cancer). Although a particularly potent cytotoxic drug, unfortunately, it is one of the most emetic of the anti-cancer drugs.

Cholecystokinin
A polypeptide hormone (33 amino acids) found at the highest levels in the duodenal mucosa (I cells). It is released by amino acids (especially essential amino acids such as phenylalanine and methionine) and long-chain fatty acids (e.g. oleic acid). The major physiological effects of cholecystokinin include stimulation of pancreatic enzyme secretion, contraction of the gall bladder, and trophic effects on the pancreas. A different molecular form of CCK — CCK-8 (C-terminal octapeptide) — is found predominantly in neurons in the enteric nervous system, where it is a transmitter.

Crohn's disease
An inflammatory lesion of the intestines of unknown cause; originally described in the ileum but now known to affect other parts of the alimentary tract, especially the colon.

Cyclic AMP
Cyclic adenosine 5'-phosphate — one of the intracellular second messengers which mediates, for example, the effects of hormones such as VIP and oxytocin and the β-receptor actions of noradrenaline.

Cyclic GMP
Cyclic guanosine 5'-phosphate — one of the intracellular second messengers which mediates, for example, the relaxation of vascular smooth muscle caused by EDRF.

Degranulation
The process by which cells

with granules containing a variety of biologically active agents release the contents of the granules to the extracellular environment. In the case of mast cells, the mediators include heparin, histamine, proteases and leukotrienes. The process of degranulation may be triggered by immunological factors, nerves, thermal stress, foods additives and insect bites (e.g. bee stings).

DIOS
Distal ileal obstruction syndrome — a similar condition to meconium ileus in the newborn, observed in older children and adults.

ECP
Eosinophil cationic protein — the most potent cytotoxic protein released by eosinophils, causing epithelial damage in the airways.

Eicosanoid
An autocoid derived from arachadonic acid (a polyunsaturated fatty acid). This group includes prostaglandins, prostacyclins, leukotrienes and thromboxane A_2.

Enkephalin (Leu- or Met-)
A small (five amino acids) endogenous peptide with agonist activity at μ and δ opiate receptors.

Eosinophilia
A condition in which there is an abnormally large number of eosinophil leukocytes in the blood.

EpDRF
Epithelial-derived relaxing factor — a putative factor released from epithelial cells which reduces smooth muscle tone; the identity of the factor has not been established.

Gastric/duodenal ulcer
A localized necrotic lesion of the gastric or duodenal mucous membrane in which the epithelium is destroyed and the deeper layers of the stomach wall may also become damaged.

Hyperaemia
An increase in the blood flow to a tissue; may occur as a result of an increased metabolic rate of the tissue (metabolic or active hyperaemia), due to, for example, an elevated activity (e.g. muscle contraction, exocrine gland secretion, increased local neural activity in the CNS) or following a period of ischaemia (reactive hyperaemia), such as may occur in muscle during intense exercise.

Hyperplasia
Any condition in which there is an increase in the number of cells in a tissue; e.g. an increase in the number of goblet cells in response to tobacco irritants.

Hypertension
Arterial blood pressure above the normal range. In a patient more than 50 years old, a value of 140/90 mmHg would be considered abnormal.

Hypotension
Arterial blood pressure below the normal range. Often occurs as a result of haemorrhage. A blood loss of 20–30 per cent produces mean pressures of 60–80 mmHg.

Hypoxia
A low oxygen content of blood or supply to tissues which is inadequate to maintain normal tissue metabolism.

IBS
Irritable Bowel Syndrome — an ill-defined disorder in which there is abdominal discomfort or pain associated with an alteration in bowel habit (diarrhoea, constipation, or alternating diarrhoea and constipation), for which no cause can be identified by routine clinical examination. Patients may have additional gastro-intestinal symptoms (e.g. nausea, early satiety, bloating, flatulence) and often symptoms outside the gut (e.g. urinary urgency, irregular periods). The pathophysiology is poorly understood but may involve disordered lower bowel motility and heightened sensitivity. IBS has been called 'asthma of the bowel' by some investigators.

Indomethacin
An aspirin-like anti-inflammatory drug originally used in the treatment of rheumatoid arthritis. It reduces prostaglandin levels by inhibition of the prostaglandin-forming cyclo-oxygenase.

Ipecacuanha
The dried root of the shrub Cephaelis ipecacuanha, *the chief constituents being emetine and cephaeline; irritates alimentary canal, causing nausea, vomiting and diarrhoea, and is therefore used as an emetic*

and also in cough medicine as a tussive agent, e.g. promoting mucus secretion.

Ipratropium bromide
An atropine-like bronchodilator used to treat asthma and bronchitis.

Ischaemia
A blood flow to a part of the body insufficient to maintain normal metabolism and hence function (e.g. contraction of cardiac muscle or CNS activity). It usually results from total or partial obstruction of an artery by a blood clot (thrombosis or embolism) or by spasm of the vessel caused by damage to the innervation (e.g. diabetes).

Labyrinthitis
A condition of inflammation of the vestibular labyrinth — the interconnecting system of cavities in the internal ear involved in the sense of balance.

MAC
Minimum alveolar concentration — usually applied to anaesthetic gases.

MAPC
Migrating action potential complex — a propagated burst of electrical activity recorded extracellularly from the muscle of the intestine. It is the electrical correlate of a propagated wave of contraction in the muscle.

MBP
Eosinophil major basic protein — a cytotoxic protein, released by eosinophils, which causes epithelial damage in the airways.

Meconium ileus
Possibly the earliest symptom of cystic fibrosis, occurring in up to 15 per cent of patients within the first few days of life. Characterized by an obstruction of the small intestine by a mass of sticky, dehydrated desquamated cells, mucus and bile. The obstruction accumulates in the foetal bowel and is normally discharged shortly after birth.

Multilobular biliary cirrhosis
A symptom of advanced cystic fibrosis — the liver and small bile ducts become blocked by inspissated (thickened) eosinophilic material which produces fibrosis and culminates in the destruction of the liver hepatocytes.

Myenteric (Auerbach's) plexus
Together with the submucosal plexus, forms the enteric nervous system; lies between the outer longitudinal and inner circular muscle and is associated particularly with the control of gut motility.

NANC
Non-adrenergic non-cholinergic — a class of neurotransmitter mechanism in addition to the classic cholinergic and adrenergic pathways. The effects may be excitatory or inhibitory on the target tissue depending on the transmitter type. Candidate inhibitory NANC transmitters are VIP, ATP and NO. SP, NK and CGRP are examples of excitatory NANC transmitters.

NEP
Neutral endopeptidase — an enzyme that degrades peptide neurotransmitters.

Neurotransmitter
A substance that is stored in a nerve ending (pre-synaptic terminal) or varicosity (autonomic) and released in response to the depolarization of the terminal by action potentials. The substance diffuses across the synaptic gap to interact with membrane-bound receptors located on the target tissue [e.g. another neuron, a muscle, an epithelial secretory cell (e.g. gastric oxynitic cell) or endocrine cell (e.g. antral gastrin-releasing G-cell)]. The neurotransmitter influences the function of the effector cell by either direct *gating of an ion channel, or* indirect *gating of an ion channel by a G-protein coupled to the generation of an intracellular second messenger such as cyclic AMP.*

Oedema
The presence of excessive amounts of liquid in the interstitial tissue spaces of the body due to increased transudation of water. The condition may be caused by increases in capillary blood pressure or in capillary wall permeability, or by a reduction in plasma-protein osmotic pressure.

PAF
Platelet-activating factor — a modified phospholipid representing the second family of autacoids derived from membrane

phospholipids, the other family being the eicosanoids.

PD
Potential charge difference across a membrane or epithelium

Peritonitis
Inflammation of the peritoneum caused by bacterial infection.

PHI/PHM
Peptide histidine isoleucine/ peptide histidine methionine — natural analogues of VIP.

Purinergic
A neuron using a purine (e.g. adenosine or ATP) as a neurotransmitter. Application of adenosine or ATP to the tissue innervated should mimic (at least in part) the response to nerve stimulation. In addition to action as a neurotransmitter, adenosine may also have a presynaptic neuromodulatory role.

RGC
Retrograde giant contraction — the single large contraction that sweeps along the small intestine back to the stomach prior to the onset of retching in the pre-ejection phase of emesis.

SCC
Short-circuit current — an index of net electrogenic ion transport, measured from the potential difference across the membrane and the resistance value (a measure of passive ionic permeability).

Sennoside
An anthraquinone laxative extracted from the dried leaflets or pods of Cassia acutifolia *and* Cassia angustifolia. *It acts as a stimulant laxative by directly activating neurons in the myenteric plexus (Auerbach's) to induce an increase in colonic propulsive motility.*

Sham feeding
An experimental technique, first used by Pavlov, whereby an animal is allowed to see, smell, taste, chew and swallow food which, instead of passing to the stomach, is transferred to the exterior through an oesophagostomy. In man, a 'modified' sham feeding technique is used, in which the subject spits out the food before swallowing. Sham feeding is used to investigate the 'cephalic phase' of control of gastro-intestinal tract secretions by the autonomic nervous system.

Spasmogen
An agent that causes muscle contraction

Sputum
The material expelled from respiratory passages by coughing, which is derived from nose, pharynx, trachea, bronchi and lung alveoli. It consists of saliva and any extraneous matter that may have entered the respiratory tract from neighbouring tissues, including mucoid secretions, desquamated epithelial cells, blood, pus and bacteria.

Submucosal (Meissner's) plexus
Together with the myenteric plexus, forms the enteric nervous system; lies between the circular muscle and the mucosa and is involved in the modulation of intestinal secretions, and fluid and ion absorption from the gut lumen.

Tachycardia
Increase in heart rate which may result from widespread influences on the heart, such as exercise, fever, emotion, hypotension or increased metabolic rate. These stimuli exert their effects by increasing the sympathetic discharge to the sino-atrial node (pacemaker) of the heart or via the release of adrenaline from the adrenal medulla.

Tachykinin
A family of peptides that includes SP and NKA.

Tetrodotoxin
A potent neurotoxin found in the gonads and other visceral structures of some fish of the order Tetraodontiformes, *such as the Japanese puffer fish. In nanomolar concentrations, tetrodotoxin selectively blocks Na^+ channels in the plasma membrane of some excitable cells, thereby preventing them from generating an action potential. Na^+ channels in nerve axons are most sensitive to tetradotoxin, whereas those in cardiac and smooth muscle cells are relatively resistant to it.*

Tussive
Irritant that stimulates cough; e.g. acetic acid.

Vertigo
A sense of instability or giddiness, often with a sensation of rotation; associated with middle-ear disease, eye disorders and cerebellar disease.

Index